AF270567

Born Sick in the USA: Improving the Health of a Nation

How healthy you are is dependent on where you live. Americans suffer more cancers, heart disease, mental illness, and other chronic diseases than those who live in other wealthy nations, despite having the most expensive healthcare system in the world. Why?

Embark on a journey to unravel the profound impact of public policies on American health from before birth in *Born Sick in the USA: Improving the Health of a Nation*. Delve into the intricate web where economic inequality weaves a tapestry of sickness stemming from a highly stressed society. This compelling read illuminates the need for transformative change in social safety nets and public policies to uplift national health and well-being. Through vivid storytelling, the book unveils the symptoms, diagnosis, and "medicine" required to steer the nation toward a healthier future. Join the movement for a healthier America by embracing the insightful revelations and empowering calls to action presented within the pages of this eye-opening book.

STEPHEN BEZRUCHKA is Associate Teaching Professor Emeritus in the Department of Health Systems and Population Health at the University of Washington. He is the author of *Nepali for Trekkers* (1991), *The Pocket Doctor: A Passport to Healthy Travel* (1999), *Altitude Illness: Prevention and Treatment* (2005), *Trekking in Nepal: A Traveler's Guide* (2011), and *Inequality Kills Us All: COVID-19's Health Lessons for the World* (2022), and contributed to *Far From the Road: A Community Health Project in the Himalayas* (2025), among other titles. He also set up a remote district hospital in the western part of Nepal and supervised Nepali doctor training there.

"A hopeful, pragmatic, data-informed guide to building a healthier future."

Sandro Galea, author of *Within Reason: A Liberal Public Health for an Illiberal Time*

"By examining the United States as his patient, Stephen Bezruchka has found a brilliant way to diagnose the serious, multigenerational health problems afflicting the country. From shortening lifespans to the emergence of chronic diseases in young people, his diagnoses are laid out in plain and powerful English. Dr. Bezruchka combines his decades of experience as a physician wandering the villages of Nepal and his teaching at the University of Washington's School of Public Health to gently but firmly deliver the truth about how the world's most expensive healthcare system makes us sick. His treatment plan would be easy and less costly, if only we can free ourselves from the delusion that the US enjoys the world's best healthcare system."

David Cay Johnston, bestselling author, Pulitzer Prize-winning investigative reporter

"An important and illuminating book, filled with disturbing facts and forensic analysis. A dangerous disease of inequality is afflicting the USA. Dr. Stephen Bezruchka offers us diagnosis, treatment, and, best of all, a preventive strategy for America's long-term health."

Kate Pickett, OBE, author of *The Good Society: And How We Get There*

"'Political medicine,' as Bezruchka calls it, is about building power to protect public health. The book itself is a great antidote to the particular sociopolitical and historical moment we face in the United States. Bezruchka draws on political and historical events, cross-national comparisons, and relatable everyday experiences – like having a baby or a bout of anxiety – to show us how health is not produced by access to health care or even good behavior, but rather by the social, political, and economic context in which we live. In moments of public health crisis, which we are most certainly in, it helps to go back to the history books and the 'old heads' who have seen it all. Bezruchka's book traces that critical knowledge to ground readers in an understanding of the complex forces that really shape our nation's health – from substance use, to maternal

mortality, and overall life expectancy. He walks us through practical steps for collective action, power building, and making a difference with strategies that are contemporary and practical. You leave the book feeling both grounded and empowered to meet the moment."
Megha Ramaswamy, Professor and Chair, Department of Health Systems
and Population Health, School of Public Health,
University of Washington

"America presents an egregious paradox – it has both the most expensive healthcare and the shortest life expectancy in the West. Bezruchka demonstrates how even the Shangri-la of universal healthcare and decreased inequality won't erase this discrepancy. Instead, he brilliantly teaches how it is baked into American individualism, capitalism, and its myths of mobility. But just as importantly, he outlines an activist pathway towards countering this toxic brew and making us healthier."
Robert Sapolsky, author of *Determined: Life Without Free Will*

"In this moment of turmoil and upheaval, the United States needs resounding clarity about what makes its population vulnerable to ill health, and what could reverse its course. Stephen Bezruchka once again provides a methodical and compelling account of how much politics, institutions, and policies, and the environments they foster, are central to our longevity and our quality of life."
Arjumand Siddiqi, Professor of Epidemiology and Canada
Research Chair in Population Health Equity, University of Toronto

"Why are Americans sicker and die younger than people in other wealthy nations despite spending so much more on health care? Drawing on decades of medical practice and cutting-edge research, Bezruchka's clear and incisive analysis reveals how extreme inequality and inadequate early childhood support have become lethal health threats. This book offers a prescription for real change which must not be ignored."
Richard G. Wilkinson, author of *The Impact of Inequality: How
to Make Sick Societies Healthier*

"Capitalism, its greatest critic showed, is full of contradictions. On one side, widely boasted, are its tendencies to improve public health as a by-product of capital accumulation. On the other side, widely denied or repressed, are its tendencies to undermine public health. This book, *Born Sick in the USA*, corrects the imbalance by systematically exploring the latter tendencies. Here is socially applied medical science that culminates in a persuasive call for action by its readers."

Richard D. Wolff, co-founder of Democracy at Work and author of *The Sickness Is the System: When Capitalism Fails to Save Us from Pandemics or Itself*

BORN SICK IN THE USA

IMPROVING THE HEALTH OF A NATION

Stephen Bezruchka

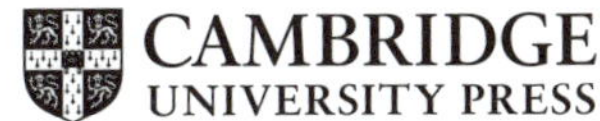

CAMBRIDGE
UNIVERSITY PRESS

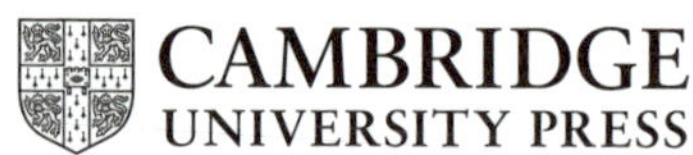

Shaftesbury Road, Cambridge CB2 8EA, United Kingdom

One Liberty Plaza, 20th Floor, New York, NY 10006, USA

477 Williamstown Road, Port Melbourne, VIC 3207, Australia

314–321, 3rd Floor, Plot 3, Splendor Forum, Jasola District Centre,
New Delhi – 110025, India

103 Penang Road, #05–06/07, Visioncrest Commercial, Singapore 238467

Cambridge University Press is part of Cambridge University Press & Assessment,
a department of the University of Cambridge.

We share the University's mission to contribute to society through the pursuit of
education, learning and research at the highest international levels of excellence.

www.cambridge.org
Information on this title: www.cambridge.org/9781009573702

DOI: 10.1017/9781009573672

First published 2026

Printed in the United Kingdom by CPI Group Ltd, Croydon CR0 4YY

A catalogue record for this publication is available from the British Library

A Cataloging-in-Publication data record for this book is available from the Library of Congress

ISBN 978-1-009-57370-2 Hardback

Cambridge University Press & Assessment has no responsibility for the persistence
or accuracy of URLs for external or third-party internet websites referred to in this
publication and does not guarantee that any content on such websites is, or will
remain, accurate or appropriate.

For EU product safety concerns, contact us at Calle de José Abascal, 56, 1°, 28003
Madrid, Spain, or email eugpsr@cambridge.org.

Every effort has been made in preparing this book to provide accurate and up-to-
date information that is in accord with accepted standards and practice at the time
of publication. Although case histories are drawn from actual cases, every effort
has been made to disguise the identities of the individuals involved. Nevertheless,
the authors, editors, and publishers can make no warranties that the information
contained herein is totally free from error, not least because clinical standards are
constantly changing through research and regulation. The authors, editors, and
publishers therefore disclaim all liability for direct or consequential damages
resulting from the use of material contained in this book. Readers are strongly
advised to pay careful attention to information provided by the manufacturer of
any drugs or equipment that they plan to use.

Contents

Foreword

As Stephen Bezruchka's book goes to print, a vast transfer of income from the bottom 99% to the top 1% is taking place in the United States. For decades, Bezruchka and his colleagues Richard Wilkinson and Kate Pickett [1] have warned about the harms to society caused by income inequality. The trends in income inequality over time have followed a reverse Robin Hood trajectory, or what the economists Anne Case and Angus Deaton [2] call a "Sherriff of Nottingham"-style redistribution. The top 1% in the United States earned 14.6% of all wages in 2021 – twice as high as their 7.3% share in 1979. Meantime, the bottom 90% received just 58.6% of all wages in 2021, the lowest share on record and far lower than their 69.8% share in 1979.

The transfer of incomes from the bottom to the top has been accomplished by breaking the collective bargaining power of unions, corporate rent-seeking, and tax cuts that overwhelmingly favor the top 1%. For clues as to who is behind these trends, we need only to look to the work of the political scientist Alexander Hertel-Fernandez [3], who has meticulously documented the influence of groups such as the American Legislative Exchange Council (ALEC), a coalition of over 2,000 (mainly Republican) state legislators, 300 large corporations, and conservative donors/activists. The avowed goal of ALEC is to disseminate "model legislation" across the US. Between 100 and 200 legislative bills sponsored by ALEC end up being enacted at the state level each year. Many of these advance the conservative agenda, including in areas such as loosening gun control, overturning climate change laws, restricting reproductive rights, passing anti-LGBT laws, overturning the Affordable Care Act, and promoting private/charter schools. But the ALEC-sponsored state laws that are most relevant to the trends described in Bezruchka's book are those that promote a Sheriff of Nottingham-style redistribution from the bottom to the top. These include state preemption of minimum wage laws and "right to work" laws that guarantee an employee's right to refrain from paying union dues or being a member of a labor union.

Much of the time, the activities of ALEC fly under the radar. When I poll students in class, I find that everyone has heard of the United Auto Workers (UAW), but almost nobody has heard of ALEC. One reason is that corporations are required by law to disclose direct campaign contributions they make to political candidates, but they are not required to disclose funding for organizations such as ALEC. The same goes for wealthy donors and activists affiliated with ALEC, who are not required to publicly disclose their support.

While wealthy Democrat and Republican donors spend about equal amounts in influencing politics, they concentrate on different goals. The Democrats focus more on influencing national politics (getting their candidate into the White House and winning House and Senate races), while Republican donors devote a whole lot more attention to state politics, where, increasingly, the action happens these days. Lest there be any doubt about the impacts of ALEC's efforts, an econometric study [4] found that, between 2011 and 2017, the introduction of state right-to-work legislation in three industries with high unionization rates at baseline – construction, education, and public administration – reduced union membership by 13% and wages by more than 4%.

Meantime, in the marketplace, the concentration of wealth in the United States is mirrored by the rise of private equity firms that are actively engaged in the redistribution of incomes from ordinary people to the oligarchy [5]. These are firms such as the Carlyle Group, Blackstone, KKR, Warburg Pincus, and Bain Capital, representing trillions of dollars of private capital in search of quick profits. Between 2005 and 2015, private equity firms focused mainly on taking over retailers such as Payless ShoeSource, Toys "R" Us, and Sears/Kmart. Leveraged buyouts are inevitably followed by aggressive cost-cutting strategies that translate to reduced pay for workers, benefit cuts, and more unstable work schedules. After retailers are saddled with huge debt loads, many of them have been forced to declare bankruptcy. During the past two decades, private equity-driven downsizing and bankruptcies are estimated to have led to the closure of 18,000 stores nationwide, as well as the loss of nearly half a million jobs. Not content with plundering the retail sector, private equity firms have been gobbling up property in distressed housing markets and driving up rents, taking over hospital and emergency rooms across the country and replacing doctors with "physician extenders," and taking over nursing homes and reducing staff ratios. A revealing statistic is that over one-third of all deaths during the COVID-19 pandemic occurred in US nursing homes, compared with 14% in Japanese nursing homes (where the majority of facilities operate as nonprofit entities) [6]. How did the Japanese succeed in holding down the proportion of COVID-19 deaths in nursing homes? Contrary to the common misconception that Japanese families are reluctant to send aging parents to nursing homes, the proportion of residents in nursing homes and residential care communities among individuals aged 65 or older is 7.8% in Japan, compared with 3.8% in the United States. The case-fatality rate among nursing home residents who were infected with COVID-19 was also comparable in the two countries (around 16%), so differences in medical care cannot explain the vast gap in nursing home deaths between the two countries. That leaves us with the explanation that the incidence of infections in Japanese nursing homes was much lower, which is, in turn, attributable to the financing of nursing homes: predominantly public, nonprofit in Japan versus private, for-profit – and increasingly owned and operated by private equity firms – in the United States. Nursing homes in Japan have higher staffing ratios, lower staff turnover, and stricter implementation of infection control protocols than those in the United States. The result is that over a million people died of COVID-19 in the United States, leading to a catastrophic 2.27-year drop in average life expectancy between 2019 and 2022. By contrast, Japanese life expectancy edged higher by 0.36 years, even in the midst of the COVID-19 pandemic.

How can we make America healthy again? One thing is clear. We cannot look to healthcare to come to the rescue. As Case and Deaton argue, our level of expenditure on healthcare has reached a point where it is itself suppressing workers' wages and causing a drag on the nation's health. The cost of healthcare coverage now amounts to 60% of the cost of hiring a low-wage worker (defined as someone earning a salary at half the median wage). Our predicament has prompted some observers to quip that

American manufacturers are now primarily engaged in the business of providing healthcare to employees; they just happen to produce other stuff (such as automobiles and widgets) on the side. As a spillover effect on the labor market, the high cost of healthcare discourages employers from hiring low-wage workers or incentivizes them to spin off low-wage jobs to subcontractors who don't offer healthcare coverage, a phenomenon known as "workplace fissuring." In short, healthcare in this country is turning good jobs into bad jobs (or eliminating jobs altogether) and contributing to the stunted economic prospects of the middle class and their poor health achievement. As the Canadian economists Evans and Stoddart [7] once remarked: "A society that spends so much on health care that it cannot or will not spend adequately on other health enhancing activities may actually be reducing the health of its population."

How can we fix income inequality? Economists tend to blame income inequality on technological change, globalization, assortative mating in the marriage market, etc., all of which sound inevitable and unavoidable. But we should never underestimate the power of wealthy individuals in diverting more income to themselves by cutting taxes, reducing social spending and weakening the power of unions. Case and Deaton argue that income inequality is not the problem per se. According to them, growing income inequality is simply the by-product of "the rigged rules by which capitalism is played out." The objective of policy should be, therefore, to punish the rule breakers (e.g. corporate rent-seekers and private equity firms engaging in predatory practices), not to redistribute income. Perhaps they have a point. But then again rigging the rules of capitalism (e.g. via political capture) would scarcely be possible in the first place without the extreme concentration of economic power.

So what is to be done? A good start is to inform yourself about the true drivers of population health and then persuade others. Bezruchka's book is a solid starting point for having this conversation. In the current polarized political climate, it might seem like a tall order to persuade those who have a different point of view. But then again, I'm reminded of the quote by Margaret Mead who said, "Never doubt that a small group of thoughtful, committed citizens can change the world; indeed, it's the only thing that ever has."

Ichiro Kawachi
Harvard University

REFERENCES

1. Wilkinson RG, Pickett K. *The Spirit Level. Why More Equal Societies Almost Always Do Better.* London: Allen Lane; 2009.
2. Case A, Deaton A. *Deaths of Despair and the Future of American Capitalism.* Princeton: Princeton University Press; 2020.
3. Hertel-Fernandez A. *State Capture. How Conservative Activists, Big Businesses, and Wealthy Donors Reshaped the American States – and the Nation.* New York: Oxford University Press; 2019.
4. Fortin N, Lemieux T, Lloyd N. Right-to-work laws, unionization, and wage setting. *NBER Working Paper Series,* No. 30098. 2022. https://doi.org/10.3386/w30098.
5. Morgensen G, Rosner J. *These are the Plunderers. How Private Equity Runs – and Wrecks – America.* New York; Simon & Schuster; 2023.
6. Abe K, Kawachi I. Deaths in nursing homes during the COVID-19 pandemic – Lessons from Japan. *Healthcare Papers.* 2021;**20**(1):78–81. https://doi.org/10.12927/hcpap.2021.26637.
7. Evans R, Stoddart GC. Consuming healthcare, producing health. *Social Science & Medicine.* 1990;**33**:1347–63.

Acknowledgments

This book began over 50 years ago when I was a medical student learning how to treat illness and injury. In a class on medicine and society, it was pointed out that, while America had been one of the healthiest nations in the 1950s, that was no longer the case.

As I show in these pages, that sad decline in our nation's health has only worsened, even though this country spends almost half of the world's healthcare budget. That's why I wrote my previous book, *Inequality Kills: COVID-19's Health Lessons for the World,* on our high rate of mortality. In this book, I consider how being sick is our pathway to an early death. In writing both books, I've gained invaluable insights and assistance from countless colleagues, friends, and others who have helped me clarify my arguments and presentation.

I gave thanks to many who led me to this juncture in the previous book. New acknowledgments are due to Youssef Azami, Mary Bassett, Georges Benjamin, Toba Bryant, Sue Carter, Esther Chung, Lilly Deerwater, Paul Ciechanowski, Sam Densen, Paul Drain, Alan Dunkin, Sandro Galea, Hilary Godwin, David Hall, David Hanscom, Lexi Lightner, Robert Lustig, Charles Mayer, Kate Pickett, Robert Sapolsky, Stephen Porges, Megha Ramaswamy, Dennis Raphael, Max Savishinsky, Mark Vossler, Don Warne, and Steven Woolf. Janice Harper has been instrumental through her editorial artfulness. Rachel Chapman has vetted my approach to race, racism, class, gender, and other forms of difference and its representation throughout the manuscript. I am grateful for her wisdom, friendship, and thoughtful elucidation. Professor Ichiro Kawachi has provided an unflinching foreword that speaks to the government's ability to shape legislation and outcomes in powerful, diabolical ways that harm us all. Anna Whiting at

Cambridge has offered extremely useful commentary and critiques. Robin Drisoll has guided the book into production. Claire Furey contributed skilled editing. Many students have helped me learn. My children, Maia and Michael, have been my greatest teachers. And my wife, Mary Anne Mercer, remains my steadfast critic and supporter.

Introduction

Healthy citizens are the greatest asset any country can have.

Winston Churchill

The United States is the only developed country without universal healthcare. Although the Affordable Care Act helped millions gain access to healthcare, we still fall short of ensuring everyone in this country can receive healthcare when they need it. But will that healthcare make us healthy? For that matter, will exercising regularly, eating healthy food, and getting our annual physicals and preventive exams help us to live longer? Mostly not. If you were born in the United States, you're already at a disadvantage compared to other rich nations. The health of people living in the United States is worse than that of people in all the other rich nations – and not because of our diets, or lifestyles, or even our limited access to healthcare. It's because we've made political choices that have placed us at the bottom of high-income countries when it comes to our health, and our lifespan.

Born Sick in the USA: Improving the Health of a Nation makes the diagnosis that our nation has misguided priorities, so we live shorter, less healthy lives. The root cause of our shorter and sicker lives is the huge economic inequality we tolerate, together with a lack of attention to our early years, when so much of our lifelong outlook for health and well-being is shaped. This is not intuitive to most people residing in the United States of America. We presume that by eating right, exercising regularly, and taking our medicines, good health is under an individual's control. To the extent that we do consider broader social factors that influence our health, we tend to focus on our access to medical care resources. Universal healthcare will give us all an equal shot at good healthcare, and thus, at health, this reasoning goes. We need universal healthcare – that is, access to quality healthcare for all people regardless of ability to pay – however, that alone won't fix the nation's health problems. Our nation's history, rooted in land expropriation, genocide, and slavery, and the pattern of political choices have more to do with the health we experience throughout our lives than any other factors.

Pointing out that the health of a nation results from political and historical factors is challenging. But as you'll read in the chapters that follow, scientific evidence has shown time and time again that America is a sick nation, and it doesn't have to be this way. We can do as well as other rich countries. Where and why are we falling short, and how can we do better?

Throughout this book I presume the reader to be a US resident (not necessarily a documented one). Your own nationality might be different. Nonetheless, because I am now an American (having been born in Canada) and largely writing this book to illuminate a critical problem in our society, I speak to the reader as a fellow American. I recognize that the word America represents a huge landmass comprising North, Central, and South America. The United States of America comprises only about 23% of that landmass and 28% of the population of the Americas. America will be used occasionally to refer to the US, but I will also use the correct terms: US, USA, United States, and the United States of America. I draw on the colloquial use of the term as it is understood here in the United States, and in other countries. This book is an appeal to the United States of America, and those who live here, to unite people, and to improve the state of our population's health.

Regarding racial designations, in concert with the Black Lives Matter movement, I will refer to people of African descent living in the US as Black, and to people of European descent as White. Both terms are capitalized to honor the weight of Black cultural continuity and surface how Whiteness functions in relationships, institutions, and communities to support systemic racism. If I refer to a study, I will use the terms used in that document.

I hope that after reading the concepts presented in the following chapters, those of us living in the US will take on the challenge of making America healthier. That we were one of the healthiest nations some 70 years ago means we can become so again. The "medicine" required is not one we will get from our healthcare system. It will require transforming the United States into a country based on principles of justice and fairness for all, not just for a few. Let's begin the healing. Be prepared for the most important lesson on health you've ever encountered.

CHAPTER ONE

Our Health in the United States

It's no measure of health to be well adjusted to a profoundly sick society.

Jiddu Krishnamurti

America is making us sick! This observation flies in the face of American exceptionalism, which has been inculcated into almost every person growing up in the United States – the view that the US is the world leader and the best at everything. We can certainly feel proud of some accomplishments. The United States has won the most Nobel Prizes, has won the most medals in the Olympics, has landed humans on the Moon, has had the most billionaires, and possesses the most powerful military in the world – the last two certainly questionable "accomplishments." But being healthy is not something we stand out in, despite spending more on medical care than any other nation by far. Healthcare represents a sixth of our total economy, over $4 trillion, or almost 18% of our gross domestic product. This is close to half of all the expenditures in healthcare worldwide. Could our medical care itself be contributing to our poor health? And might there be other factors shaping our infirmity?

I first became aware of the hazards of our biomedical care early in my career as a physician. At age 15 I had a patch of acne on the right side of my jaw. Like most teenagers with zits, I was mortified. My mother took me to a dermatologist who said, "That's no problem, we'll just radiate it." He took me to a small room, laid me on my side, adjusted a cone-shaped device above my jaw, and told me to lie still. He then left the room, closing a heavy door behind him. A brief buzzing noise like a bee about to sting followed, and the strange treatment was over. The door opened, and I left to come back again in a week for another session. After a couple of weeks of these treatments, I was delighted to have the acne disappear entirely. Ah, how wonderful! Losing my self-consciousness, I felt I had a brighter future. That was in 1958.

Seventeen years later, in 1975, I noticed a small lump where the acne had once been. Worrying about the lump, I sought medical care. The tumor was in the parotid gland, which produces saliva. I had been reassured that most tumors there were benign. The tumor and a portion of the gland were removed, and I expected to be told it was nothing to worry about. Instead, the diagnosis was lymphoma, or lymph gland cancer. I was 32 years old, and faced a grim future. I found that the 5-year survival rate for lymphoma at that time was about 65% and the 10-year only 20%. The acne cure that had brought me such relief as a teen was now laced with suffering.

My first recurrence came in 1978. Certain that I was not going to be around much longer, I changed my life course and embarked on a then little-known treatment for my kind of lymphoma. The no-treatment treatment. Research showed there was little evidence that following standard courses of chemotherapy and radiation prolonged life, so I made the decision that I would do nothing but wait and watch for ominous signs. This has now become a recognized option of treatment for my kind of lymphoma.

I received treatment only if there would be dire consequences of not doing so, such as in 1982, when a lymph node blocked my right ureter (the conduit from the kidney to the bladder) just as I was to take part in an expedition to climb Mount Everest. Radiation treatment shrunk the node and allowed me to participate in that expedition. Four members of our team were killed, and yet we reached the summit – another success that came with tragedy.

Now, as I write this, I am 82. I never expected to continue living so long. My lymphoma saga would require writing another book. Suffice it to say that I have managed to survive and thrive.

Medical care is a huge industry in the US. I have worked as a doctor here for many years, which gives me an insider's view of this immense part of the US economy. I saw that providing medical care is more of an art than a science. Until the 1960s, the scope of that art included using radiation to treat many ailments such as my acne, as well as asthma, heavy menses in women, and a range of malignancies. In what are called medical reversals, many of the treatments we used to do are no longer carried out, as they have been found to do more harm than good [1]. Acne radiation is a prime example.

At the same time, what we didn't do when I was a medical student at Stanford University in the early 1970s was give aspirin to someone having a heart attack, which is now routinely done as soon as someone complains of chest pain. In other words, our medical knowledge and our health change over time.

Younger people are increasingly suffering from chronic diseases of aging, such as arthritis, heart disease, cancers, and even dementia. We are growing old too quickly. People in other countries are not suffering from these diseases of aging at the same rate as Americans. They literally have younger, healthier, bodies.

We need to come up with a new way of thinking about how healthy we are by looking at the country we live in. You may say, "That doesn't matter. I could live in Slovenia or Sri Lanka, and so long as I eat right, exercise, and see my doctor when necessary, it's all the same. And besides, the United States has been the world leader in medical care. I wouldn't want to get sick in any other place!" This book is about showing you that is not necessarily so.

Ideas of American exceptionalism – that America and its people are singularly superior to all other countries and peoples – is instilled in Americans from the time we are born. In school we are taught to say the Pledge of Allegiance every day with our hand over our heart. "I pledge allegiance to the flag of the United States of America, and to the Republic for which it stands, one nation under God, indivisible, with liberty and justice for all." This powerful injunction is inviolable. Think of the personal freedoms underlying liberty and justice for all. Americans are free to do what they wish (within constraints). Even critics such as Noam Chomsky point out that these freedoms are not constitutionally guaranteed in most other places. Yet for all the pride this pledge, and our freedoms, instill, along with this hubris has come a distorted sense of our exceptionalism – the idea that American superiority over all other nations is divine and inherent.

I have been teaching college students since 1967 when I was a graduate student at Harvard. I then taught doctors in Nepal, and for the past 30 years, I've taught at the University of Washington. Over that long span, I sensed the resistance to any idea that counters American exceptionalism. Having been born and educated in Canada, however, I've come to see America as both a great and a flawed country. I understand that my students have been taught that everything in this country is the best, and in so many ways, America does excel. But can that be true for our health?

When you visit your doctor, she or he will measure your so-called vital signs, such as your temperature, pulse, blood pressure, weight, height, or the oxygen-carrying capacity of your blood. Hopefully your vital signs are what are termed "normal," that is, they indicate no cause for concern. Depending on how much you or your insurance company are willing or able to pay, there may follow a variety of screening tests to examine your blood and urine, and more expensive scans of your body parts. You will then be told that your health is fine and to come back in six months for another checkup. Or they might say that a blood test suggests your kidneys aren't working as well as they should. Or there is a spot on your X-ray. These days, with electronic medical records that you can access from a computer, the results are displayed as evaluated by a specialist who is paid to point out every little irregularity. You can see that information in an instant, which may cause unwarranted worry. There may be diagnoses in your record such as hypertension, diabetes, osteoporosis, or chronic lung disease. Your body needs repair, your body parts are failing, and the stress and discomfort that follow transform you. Your life changes, and so, too, does your identity. Your entire being is affected by reading medical reports of your failing health.

Yet the medical care industry does not see you and your impaired health as you experience it yourself. The medical care industry sees you as a conglomeration of cells sitting in various organs. Each of these organs has a specialist doctor who has detailed awareness of this particular body part, and there can be some value in that specialization. If these vital signs can tell us how healthy our body parts are, what might the vital signs of a country be?

Let's consider, as a thought experiment, the vital signs of a country to be the aggregate of individual vital signs. How much disease is there within a nation's borders? Most commonplace diseases are more usual in the US than in other rich nations. For example, heart disease, stroke, high blood pressure, diabetes, cancer, and lung disease are more common among Americans aged 50–74 than among those living in Austria, Denmark, Greece, Germany, Italy, the Netherlands, Spain, Sweden, and

Switzerland [2]. This is true no matter how wealthy the household is. Generally, richer folk are healthier than poorer people. However, Americans are sicker than British across the socioeconomic spectrum – richer Americans are sicker than similar and even poorer Brits [3]. Having more wealth in America still results in higher death rates than Europe [4].

Well-off US White people, those living in the richest counties, have many worse disease outcomes than people living in Australia, Austria, Canada, Denmark, Finland, France, Germany, Japan, the Netherlands, Norway, Sweden, and Switzerland [5]. In the United States there are more infant and maternal deaths, as well as worse outcomes from colon and breast cancers, childhood leukemia, and heart attacks. If you are African American, the situation is much worse. But no matter your race, gender, or economic status, you can't buy your way out of being sicker in America by living in a rich county or by having lots of wealth or by your skin color.

Given our disproportionate sickness, you might be wondering, how long do Americans live? Consider another one of a country's vital signs as how long we who reside here live, on average. Our National Center for Health Statistics reported that, in 2022, our life expectancy was 77.5 years [6]. Wow, you think, that's amazing that we live so long. But in comparison to other countries, such as Japan, Switzerland, and Singapore, where the average is almost 85 years, our longevity is not so impressive.

When I worked as a doctor in an emergency department, the nurse would measure every patient's vital signs and write them on a board for all to see. If they were within a "normal" range, I didn't worry. But if they were critically abnormal, say a blood pressure of 60/40 and a weak pulse of 150, I would immediately be alerted and be at the bedside within a heartbeat. But when do the vital signs of a country suggest immediate attention is needed?

The terms we use for these vital signs, such as life expectancy, longevity, and lifespan, require consistent definitions. Consider them for a population. Longevity, the least precise, refers to life being long-lasting. Consider human lifespan as the maximum possible length of an individual living, but this term is often used as longevity. Average length of life is commonly used to imply life expectancy. Life expectancy does not depend on the age structure of the population, namely it allows us to compare populations with a preponderance of young people with those that are predominantly older. We will further explore such vital statistics below.

Life expectancy is the total number of person-years lived by a population in a given year divided by the number of people in it. Those dying in younger years will shorten life expectancy much more than those dying at older ages. One can do a simple calculation for a population of three people. In one case, they die at ages 2, 69, and 70. There are 141 person-years, so dividing by 3 gives you a life expectancy of almost 47 years. If they died at 68, 69, and 70, then the life expectancy is 69 years. Early-life mortality impacts life expectancy considerably. I consider life expectancy the best measure of the health of a population.

Americans aren't just living shorter lives than people in other countries – we're living shorter lives each year [7]. News reports in 2022 pointed out that our life expectancy was the same as in 1996. Yet among the miracles of the last century were the vast improvements in health around the world. Declines in life expectancy outside of wars were limited to two major events. In the 1980s, HIV/AIDS devastated sub-Saharan Africa and drove down life expectancy. The other major drop was in some countries of the former Soviet Union after its breakup in 1991. Both Russia and Ukraine saw the number of deaths increase markedly. They have almost returned to their 1991 life expectancy levels. America could be facing the same challenge.

Leading public health researchers considered how many Americans were "missing" between 1980 and 2019 as a result of our death rate not being comparable to that of other countries: Australia, Austria, Belgium, Canada, Denmark, Finland, France, Germany, Iceland, Ireland, Italy, Japan, Luxembourg, the Netherlands, New Zealand, Norway, Portugal, Spain, Sweden, Switzerland, and the United Kingdom. In other words, if we had the average life expectancy of those countries over that period, there would be 11 million more Americans at the end of the last decade. For the United States, this represents 773 extra deaths each day – the equivalent of two jumbo jets crashing every day, or a 9/11 tragedy every four days [8].

So what accounts for all these extra deaths? The role of medical care in that mortal conclusion is debatable. We spend a huge amount of money on medical care, almost half of the world's total medical expenditures. Yet our health and lifespan continue to decline. Whatever we are getting for that expenditure, it isn't the best health in the world.

As these vital signs show, no matter how healthy you think you are, if you were born in the United States, your health would have been better if you had been born and brought up in many other nations. To understand this seemingly implausible statement, we explore trends in health over the last century.

HOW HAS OUR HEALTH IMPROVED IN THE LAST CENTURY?

Mortality rates in the United States fell more rapidly in the late nineteenth and early twentieth centuries than at any other period in its history. The standard of living improved immensely over those 150 years. Major health progress came from advances in sanitation as we removed fecal waste from food and water [9]. Access to clean water, through filtration and chlorination, accounts for nearly half the reduction of total mortality in major cities, and perhaps two-thirds of the decline in child mortality. We enjoyed better housing standards, pasteurizing milk led to declines in deaths from tuberculosis, and we had effective mass vaccination campaigns to avoid dying from diphtheria and other infectious diseases. Nutrition improved. Achieved stature, that is, how tall people are, showed dramatic increases toward the end of the nineteenth century in America. Americans were some of the tallest people in the world then.

In recent decades, however, our comparative height advantage has declined, consistent with our worsening health. We are now more often the biggest, the most obese, rather than the tallest [10]. What might our declining height mean? Social norms tend to favor taller men who have advantages accruing just for their height. I grew to 6 feet 5 inches. While I would like to believe that my accomplishments in life resulted from factors other than my being tall, I know my height has conferred on me a social advantage. How about looking at other measures for comparative advantages among nations?

We have discussed life expectancy, which is a commonly used measure of a country's health. Calculating life expectancy requires knowing everyone's dates of birth and of death. All rich countries have these records, and reasonable estimates exist for others. Results are published by the United Nations (UN), the World Health Organization, the World Bank, and our Central Intelligence Agency (CIA).

Another more sensitive national- or population-level health measure is infant mortality. How many deaths occur before an infant reaches age one? Increases in infant mortality, such as happened in the US from 2020 to 2022, are ominous. Maternal mortality, or deaths of women from childbirth-related causes, is another. One can consider other measures such as child or adult mortality and then look at deaths from specific causes. What can be learned from these numbers?

I coined the term "health Olympics" a few decades ago to track the ranking of countries by life expectancy. Back in the early 1950s, America could be proud of its performance in this race. The country ranked among the top ten [11].

As a medical student in 1971, I took a course from Professor Count Gibson titled "Medicine and Society." There I learned that, in 1953, the United States had the lowest maternal mortality rate of all nations. In that course it was pointed out that, by 1966, our ranking in maternal deaths had declined as other countries improved faster. This was similar for life expectancy in 1966, when the US was 12th for males and 13th for females.

My notes show infant mortality statistics where I wrote that, in 1968, we ranked 19th, while Norway ranked at the top. I noted that even removing the variable of race (given our failure to treat all races equally), we were doing poorly (i.e. we still ranked sixth). I wrote (incorrectly) that, in Mississippi, the infant mortality was higher than that of the African nation Ghana. Mississippi remains the least healthy state in America today, with its life expectancy for 2021 a little lower than that for Mongolia.

Reflecting now on those times, when the United States once had excellent mortality outcomes among nations overall, but over time that health advantage declined, I wish that this material had been stressed in my education to become a doctor. At that time, not one of the other professors ever mentioned anything about how well the US does in comparison to the health of other nations. And this is still not discussed in medical school. So what is the US' health Olympics outcome today?

In 1966, when I graduated from college, the US ranked about 13th for combined male and female life expectancy. When I went to medical school in 1970, we stood at 17th. When I went to public health school at Johns Hopkins University in 1992, we stood at 22nd. By 2022, when I began writing this book, 43 UN nations had a longer life expectancy than the United States. These include all the other rich countries and some middle-income nations such as Chile, China, Croatia, Slovenia, and Thailand, which used to have much shorter lives than we did, but have now surpassed us (see Chapter 5). Is the sky falling, or should we not be concerned with our dying younger year by year?

What should a country measure to indicate how well it is doing and whether it is making progress? Economic growth is measured and reported every month. Another supposedly important measure for a country, the gross domestic product (GDP), is the total of all goods and services produced in a country, usually expressed in dollars per person. But what does the GDP actually represent?

The concept of measuring economic growth began with Simon Kuznets, an American economist, who came up with the concept of GDP, for which he received the 1971 Nobel Memorial Prize in Economic Sciences. He also looked at the relationship of economic growth, plotted horizontally, with inequality, plotted vertically – the so-called Kuznets curve. The curve he described was an upside-down U. He postulated that, as an economy grows, inequality increases, then it reaches a plateau so that, with further growth, inequality declines, because, as workers migrate from agriculture to industry, their incomes increase, and rural workers move to better-paying urban jobs [12]. We have not yet seen that decline in inequality.

To tie economic growth to life expectancy – the health measure proposed for a country – Samuel Preston, a demographer, produced a curve in 1975 linking country per capita GDP, plotted on the horizontal axis, with its life expectancy, plotted on the vertical axis. The Preston curve shows that, starting close to zero, as a country's GDP grows, life expectancy increases rapidly. As the GDP reaches around $10,000 per capita, the life expectancy increases are more modest. At the extremes of high GDP, some countries have lower life expectancies than countries with smaller GDPs. Figure 1.1 is a curve with data for 2021 from the World Bank for GDP and UN for life expectancy.

You can see the curve bending to level off somewhere around $10,000. Dollars are adjusted to reflect different purchasing power among the countries. The United States has a high GDP, but many other countries have higher life expectancies. There is a threshold: once surpassed, economic growth no longer produces health benefits. This is counterintuitive, indeed.

Given that our life expectancy is lower than that of quite a few other nations, our focus on economic growth may not do much to produce

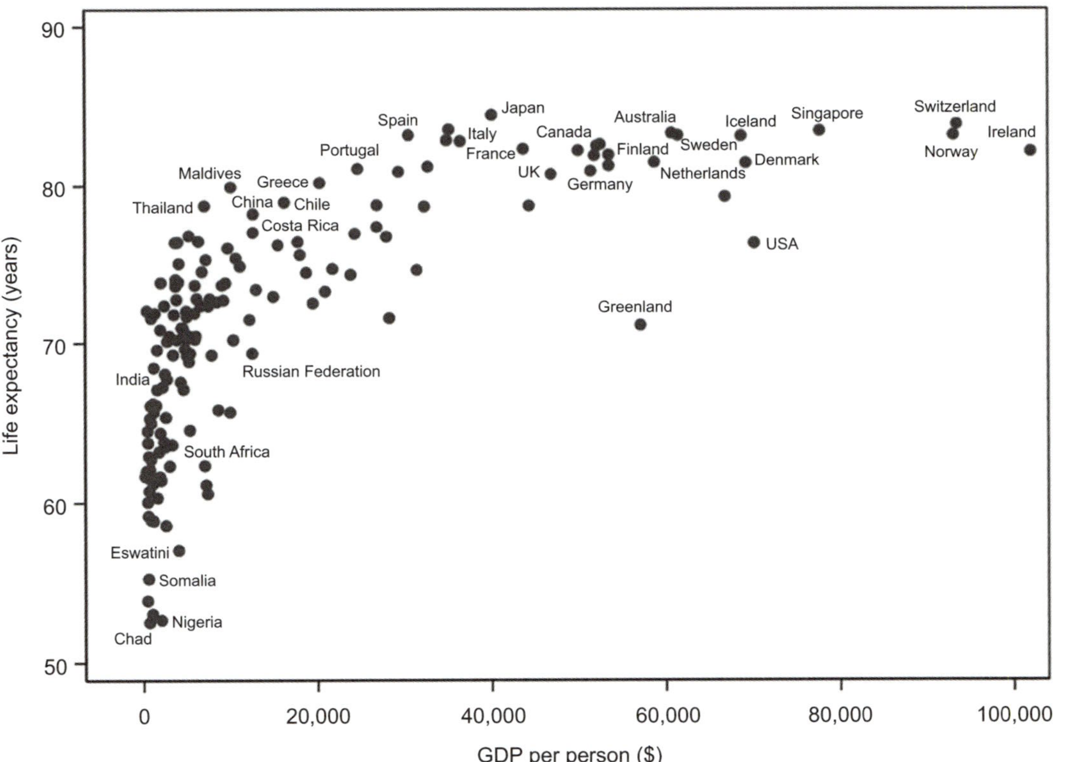

1.1 Life expectancy and GDP, 2021 (Source: Kate Pickett)

health. Japan, for example, has the longest lifespan and has had slower economic growth. Perhaps how much of our wealth we spend on healthcare determines how healthy we are? No, it doesn't. Despite all the money we have spent on healthcare, we are still far from the healthiest nation. But is living a long life really a marker of good health? After all, as the saying goes, growing old ain't for sissies. Let's consider what it means to grow old in America.

AGING ACROSS THE GLOBE

When he was 57, Ezekiel Emanuel, a bioethicist and oncologist, wrote an article titled, "Why I Hope to Die at 75" [13]. He reasons that the quality of life declines with age. He rejects the American manic desperation to extend life as long as possible. He points out that as we age there is a progressive deterioration of physical and mental functioning. Medical care has not slowed the aging process, but it may have slowed the dying process.

Many older people who suffer serious disabling conditions, such as a stroke that limits life's functions, express the desire to not live longer, as do others with many serious illnesses in old age. There is a tendency in the United States to do interventions in older people that would not take place in other rich countries with universal healthcare and salaried doctors. For example, a friend of mine requested surgery for a nonmalignant bladder tumor. He died soon after the operation from a blood clot lodging in the lung (pulmonary embolus), a common postoperative complication. My next-door neighbor died similarly after nonessential surgery. By reading obituaries of Americans, one discovers how often death occurs after some medical intervention. Yet, the for-profit medical care system in the US incentivizes such actions.

I leave it for the reader to decide if they would rather die at age 75, as Emanuel desires. If you do, you are rewarded for living in America with its low longevity. Yet some of us do live long lives, and those extra years aren't necessarily without meaning. As I write this book in my ninth decade of life, pleasure, for me, is still meaningful work. What is meaningful varies from person to person. When I was 70, I relished the additional years that I had been blessed with, despite the lymphoma, and accepted death at any time. Now I have a variety of chronic ailments in my organ recital – hearing issues, balance issues, spinal stenosis, venous insufficiency, gut problems, and atrial fibrillation, among others. While I'm not thrilled with this loss of ability from aging, I still enjoy being productive in my way. Even though as individuals we may live long and healthy lives, as a population, we have failed. But maybe what matters is reflected in the pursuit of happiness that is specified in the US Declaration of Independence. What shifts if we accept shorter lives and reflect on our pursuit of happiness?

DOES LIVING IN AMERICA MAKE US HAPPIER?

In my university courses on population health, I devote a whole class to well-being and happiness. My students note a decline in their enjoyment or pleasure or mirth. They have no disagreement when confronted by happiness measures taken from the annual World Happiness Report. That report tabulates average life satisfaction. Happiness is a subjective measure, as there is no biological parameter to indicate how happy someone is.

People in the Scandinavian countries consistently report the most happiness. For 2021–2023, the US ranked behind 22 other nations [14]. The happiness resulting from our constant pursuit of it has declined over the last few decades. The drop has been greatest among women. Older Americans report more happiness than younger people, but less than in other nations. Amidst all this lost joy, the happiness industry is telling Americans to make ourselves happy, center our joy, follow our bliss. Despite such phrases tripling in American self-help books, this advice is not working. When I was a medical student at Stanford in the early 1970s, the most popular course on campus was about sex. Today, at Yale University, the most popular course in its long history is about happiness. What accounts for happiness? Let's consider the happy Scandinavian nations and how we compare.

Reports have explored reasons for the Scandinavian nations' happiness. These include a well-functioning democracy, excellent social welfare benefits, low levels of crime and corruption, and the citizenry feeling free and trusting each other and their governmental institutions. Reasons presented for the United States not doing so well include our poor social safety net, our saturation with digital media, and having one of the world's highest levels of income inequality.

Professor Robert Lane, at Yale University, suggested that, despite Americans having more and more things and opportunities, we are less satisfied with our marriages, our homes, our work, and our financial situations [15]. We spend less time with friends, relatives, and family than we did in the past, and less than people do in other nations. We have so much information at our disposal that is supposed to make life easier and thus more enjoyable. But this is not happening. We are not happier, our lives are not easier, and they are certainly no longer or healthier than lives in many other countries. Our technology hasn't made us happier or healthier, and nor does supposedly having the best medical care in the world.

If we've failed, despite having the best medical care in the world, what we have to look at next is the role medical care plays in producing health, and the link between health and happiness. How is it we spend so much on healthcare and have so little to show for it? Is it just another outcome of the unequal access to healthcare that comes with our privatized healthcare system in the United States? Or might there be something else at work?

CHAPTER TWO

How Medical Care Impacts Your Health

Primum non nocere (First do no harm)

The Hippocratic oath

For many readers in the US, this chapter may be the most challenging of the entire book. People here typically consider medical care as the most important factor in producing good health. We spend more than any other country on healthcare. That should mean we get the most value from our expenditure. And since it is tacitly assumed that we lead the world in important matters, we should lead the world in health outcomes. The previous chapter pointed out the fallacy of our being the healthiest.

Let's begin with medical harm – the most unforeseen facts about healthcare – then follow with looking at doctors and other healthcare workers. Next we'll consider the marketing of medical care, its cost and value together with its scope, and finally consider current corporatization of the industry. This chapter is a demanding read.

The principles guiding medical care in the United States are somewhat along the lines of "Don't just stand there, do something!" Or for a surgeon, "If in doubt, cut it out." Ironically, medical care itself, even when trying not to, often causes harm. I began this chapter with the Hippocratic oath, because medical care itself, when studied, is always a leading cause of death. A few decades ago the term "medical harm" appeared to describe this situation. I can't say we have more of this medical harm in the US than other countries, but we certainly have our fair share. One estimate from Johns Hopkins University School of Medicine is that medical harm may be the third leading cause of death in the United States [16]. A report from Australia confirms the same there [17]. Astounding, right?

The first investigative reports on medical harm in the United States appeared in 1991. These led to an outpouring of research findings, personal testimonies, reports by the Institute of Medicine (now named the National Academy of Medicine), and books by doctors, lawyers, and many others. One key finding is that when doctors go on strike, morticians have less work to do. That is, deaths go down [18]. The phrase medical harm has been sanitized to patient safety, but harm it remains. Examples include leaving surgical instruments behind in the body, prescribing drugs that patients are allergic to or drug combinations with adverse synergistic effects, doing unnecessary tests and procedures whose outcomes can lead to worse health, and technical complications with various tests and surgeries. My sister-in-law taught school the day before she went for elective surgery at the top-rated hospital in Washington state. Tragically, she died on the operating table from an instrument malfunctioning. And recall my own deeply harmful acne treatment.

If the previous chapter is to be believed, we are facing a paradox when considering what healthcare does to produce health. Either healthcare does not influence the health of a country much, or the way healthcare is structured in the United States is flawed. There is evidence to support both these premises. What can be learned from exploring the role of healthcare in producing health? Let's begin with healthcare workers.

HEALTHCARE WORKERS

Being a medical doctor is an esteemed profession in most societies. Adding the title doctor before your name and introducing yourself as Doctor Jones sets you apart from others. When you write the letters MD, after your name, the two simple letters connote your status as someone special and likely raises your salary. Call those exceptional people "MDeities."

Other appellants for those who practice forms of medicine, such as DO (doctor of osteopathy), OD (doctor of optometry), DC (doctor of chiropractic), DPM (doctor of podiatric medicine), and DDS (doctor of dental surgery), carry less prestige in the United States than does the vaunted MD, while most with a PhD do not call themselves doctor outside of universities, and now on social media.

The high regard that doctors used to have has declined somewhat for the last half-century, and more recently with the rebirth and acceptance of various alternative modes of healing, together with the corporatization of the profession, with its demands for efficiency and spending less time on direct patient encounters [19], but MDs are still valued in society. This is certainly apparent from the cost and difficulties in getting admitted to medical schools in the United States. Many hurdles of entry into medical schools, such as high grades and test scores, considerable volunteer experience, and outstanding letters of recommendation, as well as high tuition costs, along with few medical schools per capita, severely limit how many doctors can practice in America. The selectivity of who gets in, and the limit to how many can practice, have contributed to the esteem we tend to hold for doctors.

Besides having considerable status, making lots of money is also a top reason for many becoming a doctor in the United States. I'm told a surgeon in Sweden doesn't make much more than a high school teacher there, while the compensation American physicians receive is the highest in the world, including for women doctors, who now make up the majority in many American medical schools. Although women doctors continue to be paid less than men doctors, the pay differential is smaller than in many other occupations. US women doctors still make more than men physicians in any other country.

One part of explaining our paradox, then, is that by making it so difficult to become a doctor in the United States, those who provide medical care become highly regarded. Doctors are also not typically from the poorer segment of society. In part, their prestige has more to do with effective medical media marketing than the actual value of such professionals. Does the value doctors provide exceed, say, the value of nurses who provide round-the-clock medical care? Why do we confer so much status on doctors, but not on nurses? Why do we value medical degrees so much more than we value graduate degrees in education, or those who risk their lives in certain skilled labor jobs, such as logging workers? Besides being an artifact of ongoing patriarchal sexism, perhaps this esteem that physicians uniquely enjoy is due to marketing.

MARKETING OF MEDICAL CARE

In the 1960s and '70s, doctors in Canada and the United States did not engage in advertising for their services, as back then, it was a violation of the ethical code. However, doctors did advertise products such as cigarettes. You've probably seen the vintage ads featuring doctors – or just men in white coats looking like doctors – who assured consumers that a certain brand of cigarette was milder and caused less irritation than competing brands. While we now know that there's nothing healthy about cigarettes, doctors now put their names on a rising number of products advertised as health promoting, and the ethical code has changed to permit them to advertise their services directly to their patients. Medical marketing is now a huge industry.

In the print media there are full-page ads, as in *The New York Times*, for a wide range of doctor groups and hospitals touting their services. Beginning in the late 1990s, and after pressure from the pharmaceutical industry, the US Food and Drug Administration (FDA) eased restrictions on pharmaceutical advertisements, permitting direct-to-consumer advertising (DTCA). As ads for pharmaceutical drugs began appearing in magazines, radio, and television, drug companies discovered that sales were much greater when their ads targeted the general public rather than reaching these same patients indirectly through doctors. Previously, drugs were marketed to doctors only in medical journals, or by drug reps. These relentless salespeople were usually attractive young women who went to doctors' offices pitching one drug or another that had a high profit margin.

The more that was spent on DTCA, the more rapid the increase in sales [20]. The drugs being pushed are not just the old standbys that have earned an indisputable therapeutic benefit, such as aspirin, morphine, and penicillin. They are often recently developed pharmaceuticals doing maintenance therapy – that is drugs that keep your blood pressure down in the normal range that must be taken seemingly forever. There are no drugs that cure high blood pressure. And there would be little incentive for drug companies to develop such cures, as maintenance therapy provides an income stream for as long as the patient lives – for example, people with chronic conditions such as diabetes, hypertension, and psychiatric disorders – which ensures ongoing profit streams. Everyone is familiar with the "ask your doctor about" format in pharmaceutical ads, whether in print, on television, or on social media sites. These ads certainly enhance the perception of the value of medical care. But few viewers pay any attention to the litany of side effects, which often include death.[1] When I ask students how they feel about these drug ads, some say, "Without these ads, how will we know what drugs to ask for?" We've gone from physicians selecting the appropriate medication based on their training and experience to patients selecting their medication based on advertisements! The United States is the only nation worldwide with such an aggressive form of drug marketing, and in a profit-driven medication industry, the ads work.

But marketing cannot improve disease management. Studies with actor patients show that if you go to a healthcare worker with symptoms of something for which a drug may be beneficial, but don't ask for a specific drug, you are less likely to get that drug than if you just go to your doctor and ask for it directly. In today's fast-paced office visits, it is quicker for the harried physician to just provide what is asked for and move on to the next patient. Such is the assembly-line work of providing healthcare in the United States.

Another form of advertising is biomediatization, where news reports are more about advertising some procedure or medical product that has become available than they are about providing factual and unbiased content. Such "news" substitutes for having to pay for promotion. Let's dissect medical care.

COST AND VALUE OF MEDICAL CARE

Medical care is highly valued in the United States. But does that justify its high cost? We're all familiar with the astronomical medical bills patients receive, such as "facility fees" of up to thousands of dollars that can be charged to patients by hospitals they never even went to – because the physician they saw was associated with that hospital. Hospitals can now even charge for "skin-to-skin" contact for just letting a father hold his newborn baby! And you've undoubtedly been surprised by the high charges for over-the-counter medications when delivered in a hospital setting. A single baby aspirin can cost anywhere from 65 cents to $18 if provided in a hospital. These egregious charges should be questioned, but mostly they aren't. Unlike most items you purchase in a market, you have no idea of the price you will be charged, because there is no set menu

---

[1]   Search for the spoof ad for Progenitorivox, which I have my students watch.

of charges. You aren't given many options regarding your care, and the bills don't arrive until months after the care is delivered.

That still doesn't answer why we spend so much on medical care and receive, in return, so little value in terms of better health. To begin with, the economic system that runs medical care in the United States tries to maximize profits. Being treated in a for-profit institution produces worse health outcomes than when there is no profit motive [21]. Yet we've been led to believe that medical care in America is so expensive because it is far better than cheaper care elsewhere. Consider the many political debates about whether we should have universal healthcare in the United States. Inevitably, the medical care in countries such as Canada or England are pointed to as having inferior forms of healthcare by those who oppose healthcare as a human need.

The term financial toxicity initially referred to the personal costs of cancer treatment in the US. The National Cancer Institute has a whole website devoted to such pecuniary distress. The high costs of cancer care lead to patients forgoing getting their medical prescriptions filled, borrowing more money, becoming anxious or depressed and reducing their spending on food and other necessities, catalyzing a downward health spiral. This dilemma is not limited to cancer care in America. It's no wonder then that medical care is one of the biggest causes of bankruptcy in the US, even for insured patients, something unheard of in other rich nations.

The concept of healthcare insurance began in the United States as accident insurance at the end of the nineteenth century. This insurance provided compensation for railroad and steamboat accidents. Sickness coverage began soon afterwards, followed by disability insurance, to replace lost wages. Before this, one had to pay for medical services out of pocket. We then got healthcare insurance. I use the term healthcare insurance and not health insurance because healthcare does not do that much for health. Calling it health insurance distracts us from understanding what produces health in a society, and implies that we are insuring being healthy. Not so.

The first attempt to have an optional public healthcare insurance system was proposed by President Truman in 1945. The American Medical Association, among other powerful guilds, denounced this as socialism. Instead, healthcare insurance was typically offered as a part of what you received at a job – employer-sponsored insurance won through union activism. Part of the reason was to provide additional benefits to workers since wage controls were imposed by the government during World War II to avoid siphoning workers away from the war effort.

Consolidation of hospitalization insurance led to Blue Cross and Blue Shield systems, initially not-for-profit, which nevertheless evolved to become extremely profitable enterprises. There followed Medicare, hospital insurance for those over the age of 65, and Medicaid, for people living below the poverty level, by 1965. Medicare expanded to cover services for those with certain disabilities and for end-stage kidney care. The kidney became the first, and only, insured human organ in America. Medicaid plans varied from state to state. As costs of medical care soared, presidential administrations sought to develop universal insurance systems, beginning with President Nixon, then President Clinton. But fierce opposition from the medical insurance industry doomed the plans.

When various government expenditures for medical care are added up in this country, we have already spent more for medical care than countries with universal healthcare. Our government spends enough so that everyone could have healthcare without having to pay for it out of pocket. So, why not have a single-payer, universal healthcare system?

President Obama successfully got a limited healthcare insurance plan enacted. While there were demands for a single-payer system so everyone had insurance, Obama said this option was "off the table." His administration felt that a single-payer system was politically unachievable, as the incredibly profitable healthcare insurance industry did not want to lose its cash cow. The Patient Protection and Affordable Care Act, also known as the Affordable Care Act (ACA) or Obamacare, came into effect in 2014. The ACA prohibited insurers from discriminating against or charging higher rates for individuals based on preexisting medical conditions, and ensured that they must now offer a standard set of coverage. With the passage of the ACA, nearly 40 million more Americans could access medical care than before. Despite the advent of the ACA, however, as we pointed out in the previous chapter, our life expectancy as a measure of health has continued to decline. This decline is consistent with access to medical care not being the most important factor in improving health. This surprising fact was first demonstrated with Medicare, which was enacted in 1965 and came into effect in 1966. No mortality improvements could be attributed to Medicare coverage for the subsequent 10 years [22]. The main benefit of Medicare was economic – namely, fewer out-of-pocket costs to seniors.

Despite all the progress in offering medical care services at a lower cost, a large fraction – close to a third – of the US population still has limited or no access to medical care. At the same time there have been serious attempts to repeal the ACA. The political denouncements of universal healthcare have worked. Access to healthcare is not considered a right in the United States.

As pointed out in Chapter 1, if we consider the gains in health over the past few centuries, the fact that we are living so much longer than we did 100 years ago mostly did not come from medical care. Our use of language confuses us. We say we "access health" and "get health" and "insure health" and "pay for health," but I propose it is more accurate to say health*care* instead of health in these cases. We are led to believe it is healthcare that produces health. Do you want healthcare or do you want health?

Health system is another misleading phrase used widely. The term implies there is a structure in place to produce health and commonly refers to what countries have set up. We are in fact speaking of healthcare systems. For a systematic approach to producing health, perhaps only Cuba, with its social and economic supports, can speak of having a health system. Tiny Cuba has been portrayed to Americans as a major threat to the United States, and the country has been blockaded for more than half a century so as not to let their socialist concepts succeed, or worse yet, seep into our populace as a positive model. Despite this hardship, Cuba's health is on a par with the United States, whose standard of living greatly eclipses Cuba's.

Although we enjoy a vastly improved standard of living than in the past, there remain extreme inequalities of access. Take, for example, sanitation. We have structured society to be more hygienic by separating fecal and other human and animal waste from food and water. We don't think about this process, as it is done by the cities and towns where we live through modern plumbing, sewage disposal, and water treatment. Yet there remain several million dwellings in this country that do not have clean water piped into homes or effective disposal of human waste. Consider Flint, Michigan, a once-thriving hub of the auto industry, where over two-thirds of its residents are Black. When its water source was changed from Lake Huron to the Flint River in 2014 to deal with a financial crisis and provide a cheaper service, residents were exposed to toxic chemicals, and lead poisoning levels, especially among children, skyrocketed throughout the county. This constituted a federal public health emergency. Just one hour away, however, in affluent Grosse Pointe, Michigan, where nearly 98% of the residents are White, the water piped into residents' homes comes from Lake St. Clair, and is just fine.

SCOPE OF MEDICAL CARE

Are *we* treated with medical care? Not exactly. More accurately, medical care treats our parts. We are made up of cells that are arranged in our organs such as the heart, lung, kidneys, and muscles. Mostly medical care treats cells and organs. You may take aspirin to make your platelets (cells in the blood) less sticky so you don't have a heart attack, statins that affect your liver cells to control your cholesterol, and another category of drugs called selective serotonin reuptake inhibitors (SSRIs) (one of which is Prozac®) to treat brain cells. Most of the pharmaceuticals we consume work on cells. Medical care also treats organs, such as the heart. So when you have a blockage in an artery feeding the heart muscle – a heart attack – you typically have that clot removed by a cardiologist so the heart muscle can receive oxygen and glucose. If you have an inflamed appendix, that organ will likely be removed by a surgeon. And so on.

Medical care does not treat the whole individual human. If it did, when a homeless man came into my emergency department with a complaint of belly pain, I would evaluate him medically, spending thousands of dollars in investigations, to see if he required admission to the hospital. But that was not what typically happened. If he did not need immediate admission to the hospital, I had to send him back on the street, regardless of his pain or need for warm food and housing. If the nurses were cooperative, he might get a meal.

If medical care treated the whole person, a sick person with no place to go would be provided with a comprehensive medical exam, and given a home, nourishment, and meaningful work, together with social support. Alas, that treatment is not in the hospital formulary. And being homeless is only listed in the massive *International Classification of Diseases* (ICD) compendium as a factor "influencing health status or contact with health services" – a social determinant.

All diseases have two causes: one biologic or pathologic and the other social. Medical care in the US focuses on the former, but wholly disregards the latter. Not so in many other countries. In Canada, for example, medical care includes social prescribing. This means not just treating the diagnosed disease, but attending to the social circumstances as well. The unhoused man with pain, whom I described above, could be prescribed food and meaningful work, as well as housing. But lacking an integrated biosocial approach, and, instead, providing profit-driven interventions, medical care in the US increasingly relies on efficiency – and what could be more efficient than prescribing drugs? Yet many of the drugs we prescribe either create more health problems (termed "side effects") or are no more effective than doing nothing, especially when the individual prescribed them does not have guaranteed shelter, food, access to clean water and sanitation, or protection from violence.

What about "lifesaving drugs" you might ask? Consider statins, cholesterol-lowering drugs, for cardiovascular disease. Studies show that their use prolongs life by around ten days [23]. Similar research shows that treatment for congestive heart failure, a condition related to economic inequality that we will explore in Chapter 5, postpones death by around a month [24]. I'm not suggesting you stop taking your medication; instead, I'm shifting the discussion from the need to treat the *disease* to treating the *origins* of disease. Consider diabetes, a disease that can often be controlled individually with medication. But is medication the answer to controlling diabetes nationwide?

Diabetes wasn't common in the past, but has become an important disease around the world. As acute diseases associated with poor sanitation declined, chronic diseases associated with sedentary lifestyles and diets high in sugar and salt rose, leading to rising rates of diabetes and cardiovascular disease. We have replaced diseases of young bowels with diseases of old arteries.

Diabetes produces many arterial afflictions. Diabetes affects how the body processes glucose, the main energy substrate driving bodily functions. Much of the food you eat is converted into glucose, which enters the bloodstream to feed your cells and organs. Insulin, a hormone released from the pancreas when glucose rises in the blood, enables glucose to get into cells, and thus provide energy for the cell or organ (composed of cells) to do its job.

There are two kinds of diabetes, types 1 and 2. In type 1 (also called juvenile-onset diabetes), the pancreas doesn't produce enough (or even any) insulin for the tasks required. Type 1 diabetes develops in young people. In 1921, Frederick Banting and Charles Best injected insulin extracted from cows, and then pigs, caged in slaughterhouses into people with diabetes, heralding insulin as a lifesaving treatment for diabetes. They chose to not patent the drug so that everyone could have it, and Banting received the 1923 Nobel Prize in Physiology or Medicine.

In the past, people with type 1 diabetes would monitor how much glucose was spilling into their urine to gauge how much insulin was needed to metabolize the foods they'd eaten. The process has become more automated, with monitors and pumps almost replacing the pancreas. With good control of glucose, the myriad side effects of diabetes lessen. People with diabetes can live pretty normal lives.

The more common type 2 diabetes, also called adult-onset diabetes, results from the body producing insulin but not being able to utilize it effectively. Blood glucose rises. Treatments vary from diet and exercise to various drugs to help utilize insulin. Type 2 diabetes may arise from our inactivity coupled with consuming huge amounts of sugar, mostly from a diet heavy in highly processed foods. Consider this the nutrition transition. With the advent of agriculture, we went from a period of under-nutrition to one of urbanization, economic growth, and consumption of processed foods. As we consumed more fats and sugar in these processed foods to help us deal with the stress of society, obesity emerged. Such changes, especially in early life, have led to type 2 diabetes being ubiquitous around the world.

A 2021 report to the US Congress on using federal programs to prevent and control diabetes from the US Department of Health and Human Services pointed out that, in 2018, 1 in 10 Americans had diabetes and 1 in 3 was in a prediabetic state [25]. The 2017 costs of this disease were estimated to be *a third of a trillion dollars*. For prevention they recommended increasing breastfeeding rates (including having paid maternity leave to make this possible for working women), reducing consumption of sugar-sweetened beverages, and improving the physical environment to facilitate exercise. They recommended addressing the social determinants of health (SDOH) (to be discussed in Chapter 3). Drug treatment has limited benefits compared with treating the social determinants via social prescribing. There is no drug to counter the effects of impoverishment, stress, being unhoused, and other socioeconomic factors that cause and maintain diabetes.

Type 2 diabetes has especially increased among US Black youth. Black people are more than twice as likely to develop diabetes in the US than White people [26]. Higher rates of low birthweight among Black infants are one cause. Another cause is that, due to political, social, and economic disenfranchisement, many Black communities suffer food apartheid – the systemic and intentional food-access disparity where stores do not offer many or any healthy foods. The stress and violence of racism is another social determinant underlying high rates of diabetes. This rise in diabetes, combined with racial inequities blocking access to health services, screening, and timely, quality treatment, and racial bias in medical care if access is gained, leads to many more diabetes-related complications among African Americans as they age, including blindness, amputations, atherosclerosis, and kidney disorders.

Drug treatment for type 2 diabetes is not that effective. An old standby – metformin – is considered the most valuable and is commonly prescribed. Metformin, long off patent, is not expensive, and, therefore does not generate big revenue, so it is not marketed. Readers see drug ads for many new expensive drugs to control diabetes that are of less benefit, but are more profitable for the pharmaceutical industry.

The contemporary increase in diabetes over the last 50 years relates to early life issues. Consider a natural experiment. Instead of researchers setting up a study to understand a phenomenon, they look at health-related events that happened in the past to a given population. During World War II in the Netherlands, from November 1944 to April 1945, daily rations were cut to 1,000 calories. Pregnant women were supposed to get extra food, but often didn't. Those women were followed to see what happened to the infants they birthed. Those infants, whose time *in utero* was nutritionally and psychologically stressed, were more likely to develop diabetes as they aged [27]. When these female infants became adults and had their own babies, without those nutritional stresses, they too developed diabetes in adulthood. We will see later how stresses such as these can affect subsequent generations through epigenetic means.

Studies show that infants born with a low birthweight are more likely to develop diabetes as they age [28]. Low birthweight points to impaired growth of the fetus, which can contribute to insulin resistance in adults, namely the inability to use the body's own insulin, leading to type 2 diabetes. Those born of low birthweight who gained considerable weight in their first year of life typically became obese as adults and were especially prone to diabetes. This finding represents the fetal origins hypothesis, namely that many adult diseases were programmed in the fetal period. This will be further explored in Chapter 4.

Consuming sugar may be a stress reliever in the short term, but it affects diabetes at a population level, as well as your individual health [29]. Countries with more obesity have higher rates of diabetes. Does increased sugar consumption, independent of its link to obesity, cause diabetes? Maybe, but the evidence is not uniformly accepted. Nonetheless, consuming lots of sugar is not good for you, a concept that will be explored in Chapter 6.

Healthcare should treat not just individuals, but also populations, even countries. But so far, it does not. Taking life expectancy as our measure of health, let's consider what the relationship is between our lifespan and how much money a country spends on healthcare. Figure 2.1 shows length of life for 10 rich countries and the amount they spent per capita on healthcare from 1995 to 2015 [30]. The dollar amounts are adjusted for purchasing power parity, namely, the dollar amount presented there can buy the equivalent amount of goods in each of the countries. Notice the curve for the United States. Back in 1995, the life expectancy for Japan was greater than the US had in 2015. It seems that the best we could do was pretty shameful. Japanese people have the longest lives of any nation and spend comparatively little on healthcare.

Modern medical care in the United States can avert only about 10% of mortality [31]. But that is not what is commonly believed [32]. Instead, we are told we have the best healthcare in the world, so we must be the healthiest people in the world. Even for conditions that can be effectively treated by medical care, such as heart attacks, appendicitis, cancers, and various forms of trauma, the US does poorly compared with other nations. The American-based Commonwealth Fund tracks the research regularly.

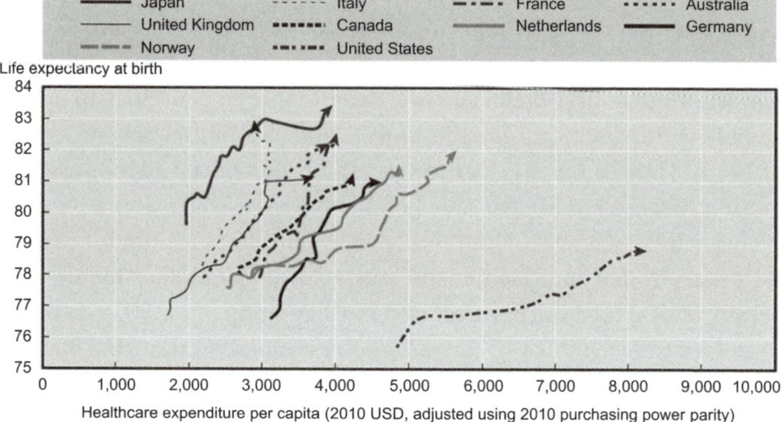

2.1 Healthcare expenditure and life expectancy gains from 1995 to 2015 for Australia, Canada, France, Germany, Italy, Japan, the Netherlands, Norway, the United Kingdom, and the United States [30].

Looking at such avoidable deaths, and how much those deaths have been reduced over 10 years in several countries, the United States stood the worst and had the smallest reduction from 2009 to 2019 [33]. Whatever we are doing with our healthcare system, it is not working well when compared with those of other countries.

Most people presume this disparity is due to our lack of universal healthcare, but what are the impacts on health of universal healthcare, Medicare for All, and single-payer healthcare (all meaning that everyone has access to medical care), and what do those impacts reveal? The evidence suggests that access to healthcare itself has less effect on a nation's overall health than one might think.

One study tracked healthcare use in Winnipeg, Canada, from 1986 to 1996. Everyone had access to healthcare. During this period the province cut costs of medical care by limiting unnecessary use of hospital beds. They tracked medical care usage by people divided into fifths (quintiles) of income. Days in hospital were highest for the lowest-income fifth over this period, with decreases in stays over the decade. Mortality rates dropped as well. They observed that the greater the decline in healthcare services, the greater the improvement in mortality. In other words, the less healthcare people had, the longer they lived. The researchers concluded that universal healthcare alone, though a necessary human right and resource, was not effective in improving population health or reducing inequalities in health in the absence of other major social and political changes [34].

This finding is not an outlier. Most studies on the impact of access to healthcare show that other SDOH, especially the meeting of basic needs, social entitlements [35], social expenditures, and social prescribing, matter more in addressing population-level disparities in health. What these studies tell us is that economically marginalized people need more than greater access to healthcare in isolation of improved access to other resources and improved living conditions. Since the US has more income inequality, a greater lack of social safety nets, and more impoverishment of its most vulnerable populations than any other rich country, these are other reasons why medical care's effectiveness is limited on its own. It makes sense that the children of impoverished parents in the lowest income brackets suffer worse outcomes from medical interventions; this is due to many factors, such as their lack of rights and resources (including food, housing, and work), income insecurity, and their exposure to environmental racism and institutional, including medical, violence.

Take pediatric heart transplants, a remarkable technical procedure that can save lives in infants and children with congenital heart damage. A study at the Boston Children's Hospital showed that there is greater rejection of the transplanted heart in children living in low-income families in neighborhoods that are underserved and underresourced regarding healthcare [36]. They speculated on reasons being biological and asked for confirmation in further studies. Subsequent multicenter studies demonstrated rejection among Black pediatric patients regardless of social class and access to healthcare services [37], suggesting that racism and impoverishment stress the body in similar ways, make postoperative care difficult, and endanger survival. In the United Kingdom this relationship between poverty and organ rejection in the short term was not seen. There is more social support and welfare benefits to those of limited means in the UK. For all adult heart transplants as well, there is a greater chance of rejection for those in the United States than for those in England [38]. This is consistent with disease outcomes being worse in the United States than in England [3].

Given these findings, should we abandon the movement for universal healthcare for all in the US and eschew medical care altogether? Absolutely not. We need quality medical care to do what it can do best – treat illness and injury. That care should be available to all without having to pay money at the point of service delivery. Studies show that primary care – the care delivered by family doctors, nurse practitioners, physicians' assistants, primary care internists, and pediatricians – is the most effective part of medical care [39]. Sometimes we need specialists in neurosurgery, endocrinology, or orthopedic surgery. But most problems can be addressed by primary care. What is required is ease of access to that care and developing a long-term relationship with a single practitioner, rather than having a succession of specialists who parade around the patient over time, each caring for a different organ. Yet there are few primary care practitioners (PCPs) in proportion to specialists working in the United States, and their numbers are decreasing. Burnout is common and the pay lower. Most medical students prefer esoteric specialties, which offer more income, status, and competence in doing one thing well.

The paucity of PCPs contributes to our poor health outcomes. Within the US, the higher the proportion of PCPs, the lower the mortality, especially from heart disease, cancers, and lung disease. However, their number, together with the lower proportion of primary healthcare expenditures, has declined considerably over the last few decades, and this contributes to the worse outcomes this country has in comparison to others [40,41]. This financial neglect of primary care is sickening us and is killing us.

CORPORATE TAKEOVER OF MEDICAL CARE

Another factor leading the decline of our healthcare system is the corporatization of medical care. Fewer and fewer healthcare doctors have their own offices and practices. They are now employees in the medical–industrial complex, a term coined by Barbara and John Ehrenreich in 1970, who argued that healthcare should be a democratic exercise. Instead, the industry has grown considerably. I first encountered this expansion in 1980, when our emergency medicine group had to undertake our own billing for the services we rendered outside of what the hospital charged. We contracted with a company that hired nurses to make the charges as high as possible, since the company received a portion of the amount billed. We couldn't lower the bill for those less able to pay inordinate amounts. Such billing companies have since become routine.

Private medical practices increasingly merge into groups. In the last decade, large corporations have been buying out these practices and hospitals. Some, such as the Sisters of Providence and Franciscans, may sound benevolent, but providing medical care has become more of a profit-driven or vulture-based service than a healthcare service. The corporatized world has required doctors, nurses, and other staff to see more patients in less time. This patient overload may lead to more medical harm. It also causes moral injury, as idealistic workers suffer from what soldiers experience after returning from the battlefield – posttraumatic stress disorder (PTSD). Increasingly common, PTSD is often characterized as "burnout" and causes many (some estimates suggest one in five) to leave careers in medical care [42]. Burdensome electronic medical records, whose major purpose is to facilitate billing, together with patient satisfaction surveys, contribute to their chronic stress. The exodus of healthcare workers has strained work for those remaining. As with combat veterans, the rate of suicide among practicing doctors is said to be twice that among active-duty soldiers. They often see themselves as scapegoats for the for-profit care system and internalize their patients' problems [43].

This profit-driven healthcare industry, a sixth of our total economy, leads to a monopolistic corporate conglomerate. Private equity funds, which attract rich investors and are mostly not transparent, become the drivers of extreme profits by cutting costs and marginalizing services. But as we've seen, healthcare services impact only about 10% of mortality. Chasing higher profits will not improve our health outcomes but, instead, worsens them.

As they take over more medical care practices, private equity funds act as vulture capitalists, degrading and consolidating the practices they accumulate, further cutting costs and increasing profits [44]. Others such as UnitedHealth Group, based in Minnetonka, Minnesota, but incorporated in the state of Delaware (for its lavish corporate-friendly tax breaks), is present in every state and is among the world's 10 largest companies.

In the 2023 Fortune Global 500 list, UnitedHealth Group ranks right up there with Amazon and Apple. They have two distinct businesses, Optum and UnitedHealthcare. Optum recently bought out the polyclinic where I had been receiving my medical care. This merger has resulted in many dissatisfied doctors leaving. Despite antitrust efforts, the legal process is allowing UnitedHealth to proceed with various mergers.

Given the enormous costs of American healthcare and its poor quality as evidenced by the harms it creates, expect further deterioration in effective care for those conditions where healthcare has the capacity to influence outcomes. So what can we do to wrestle back some control over our healthcare system?

Healthcare worker strikes are one way to gain some bargaining power. Nurses, and now even doctors, are striking, as they see themselves as essential workers just like firefighters and those working in prisons, meatpacking plants, and schools. "Work to rule" (not doing more than the minimum required) is another form of protest, used by healthcare workers in parts of Europe.

We are, thus, faced with a huge conundrum. By living in the United States, we are sicker than people in many other countries. And we cannot blame our high rate of sickness on the quality of our medical care, nor even on our relatively limited access to that care, compared with other countries with guaranteed universal medical care. Medical care, at best, has only limited effects on our health and the health of a country. We've considered the wrong question in understanding why American health is not outstanding. Rather than asking how we can receive *more* medical care, we need to ask: What does produce good health in a society? In the following chapters, we explore that question.

CHAPTER THREE

What Makes You Healthy?

Good health is not something we can buy.
However, it can be an extremely valuable savings account.

Anne Wilson Schaef

Curiously, humans are almost the only species of primates with whites in their eyes. Why might that be important? One theory is that newborns have relatively poor vision. They can see contrast best. Two contrasting items that are important for newborns are the darkly pigmented areolae of the breasts (nipples become quite dark with birth), and the white sclerae (the white part of our eye), next to the darker iris and pupil. A newborn needs to find the nipples for sustenance, and to gaze at the nourisher's eyes for assurance. Eye contact with a human is an important step in developing attachment with that person. Most of us can remember or visualize the eyes of our mothers. John Bowlby, a British psychiatrist studying orphans after World War II, found that having a single pair of eyes in front of the orphan for the first year of life presaged better development than an infant seeing many eyes or no eyes.

From our conception to when we are able to form our first memories, we live in our primal state, doing nothing to be healthy. Being mammals, we are nourished by our mothers' breast milk. There are individual exceptions, of course. Some human mothers cannot produce sufficient breast milk, or choose not to nurse, and historically there have been women who were not supposed to nurse their babies and hired so-called "wet nurses." Typically, women of the aristocracy and nobility had their children wet-nursed by women of lower status who had recently given birth. In the United States during the slavery era, enslaved Black women were forced to wet-nurse the children of those who enslaved them. Breastfeeding can still be socially uncomfortable for many mothers in the United States. Our failure to provide new mothers with paid maternity leave has made it more difficult for working women to nurse their children. The widespread availability of infant formula, a less satisfactory alternative to breast milk, has also contributed to a decline in breastfeeding.

We know that infants who are nourished on breast milk receive better nutrition and develop stronger immune systems than those who are not breastfed. Prolonged breastfeeding is associated with lower rates of adult obesity and diabetes and higher scores on intelligence tests [45]. Maternal benefits include lower rates of breast and ovarian cancers and diabetes. As with many statements in this book, we are talking about outcomes for populations or large groups of individuals. They do not translate to what happens to a particular individual mother and her infant in terms of whether or not the infant is breastfed and whether this harms or helps that particular child. Policies in the US, such as a lack of paid maternity leave, discourage prolonged breastfeeding. Most mothers wean their infants completely within the first three months.

Humans are born helpless. While some animals such as butterflies or snakes are considered independent at birth, humans are totally dependent on others for our basic needs for many years. Typically, the mother who provided breast milk as initial sustenance carried on this practice for a year or longer. The World Health Organization (WHO) advises exclusive breastfeeding for six months and extending with food supplementation for two years. Decades ago in Nepal, I would often see three- or four-year-old children still suckling. Breastfeeding is not only more nutritious, but it can be a comforting practice for both the baby and the mother. Yet exclusive breastfeeding for even six months is not the typical American routine and is more common in low-income countries than in richer ones [45]

Prior to World War II, this prolonged period of nursing was manageable, at least for upper-middle- and upper-class American White women, who were responsible for their infants' care, while their husbands worked outside the home (for Black women, there was less opportunity to stay home with their children, as the no or low wages for Black men had always meant that many Black women worked outside the home, especially in the service sector). As more American women entered the paid labor force during and after World War II, however, the gendered division of labor changed. Now, with women's access to professional jobs more possible, and greater economic instability and a higher cost of living requiring both parents to work in most households, the typical mother returns to work a few weeks after giving birth. It's no surprise, then, that breastfeeding and caring for a newborn have become more challenging.

The social policies any country enacts strongly affect a neonate's early life. Most nations grant a substantial period of paid parental leave to allow mothers and fathers to take care of their babies [46]. Sweden, for example, requires families to take paid time off work to care for infants [47,48]. Parents there are entitled to 480 days of paid parental leave when a child is born or adopted. If there are two parents in the family, each is entitled to half of those days, and 90 days are reserved exclusively for her or him, meaning that, if not taken, they can't be transferred to the other partner. A single parent gets the full 480 days. Fathers there take about 30% of all the paid parental leave. Canada, geographically closer to the US than Sweden, has a variety of policies with slightly different lengths and payments, depending on the province where you live. These programs come out of the national government employment insurance policy with maternal and paternal benefits. The minimum employment insurance maternity leave in Canada is 15 weeks, which can begin 12 weeks before the due date and can end as late as 17 weeks after birth. Parental leave can be as high as 78 weeks, and payouts vary among provinces, but can be up to 70% of earnings. Taking this leave is not risky either, as a parent's job is secure in any case. As an added incentive, employers in Canada often add to the payment received.

But for parents in the US, the opportunity to stay home with a newborn is limited. The United States is one of only two countries worldwide that does not have a nationally mandated paid maternity leave policy. The 1993 Family and Medical Leave Act grants pregnant women working in certain conditions (such as for a company with more than 50 employees, and if she has been there a year or more) 4 months of *unpaid* leave. Her job is secure for only that period of time – if she chooses to extend her leave, she can be fired. Few women can afford to be off work with no pay for four months. So it's no surprise that most women return to work a few weeks after delivering their baby. The United States is in an exclusive club. There is only one other country with a population of at least a million that does not offer paid maternity leave – Papua New Guinea, half of a big island north of Australia [49].

Fortunately, several states have passed a paid leave policy, with most offering no more than 12 weeks paid leave, with varying payments. This is a start, but to be healthy, we have evolved to require much more support in early life. Ironically, as we've entered the modern era, we've lost such support, and our health has worsened as our technology has improved. What's wrong with this picture?

PREHISTORY AND HISTORY OF HEALTH

We evolved as a distinct species in the hominin family some 500,000 years ago during the Paleolithic period. For most of that time, we lived as hunter-gatherer or forager-hunter bands, typically numbering fewer than 100. Such societies have been the most successful, longest, human adaptation on Earth [50].

In a band of fewer than 20 people, everyone knew everyone else. They worked together to obtain their food. They ate and slept together. Cooperation was essential. These bands were also egalitarian. Power was shared between men and women, and neither patriarchy nor poverty existed. While women provided the majority of calories through foods they foraged nearby, men obtained the prized meats. After a successful hunt, the meat was distributed equally. Vigilant sharing was the norm. If anyone got a smaller portion, it would be the hunters, as they could always get more. Skeletal evidence demonstrates that these people were relatively healthy.

Beginning about 10,000 years ago, a transition, the Mesolithic, gave way to the Neolithic. Human groups became more sedentary, and began to take up agriculture. Farming developed over different time periods. Plants (primarily wheat and barley) were domesticated in the Fertile Crescent (from the Eastern Mediterranean to the Persian Gulf) 9,000 years ago. Growing rice in East Asia followed, and in Central America, people planted maize, beans, and squash. In Northern Africa, pastoral societies began domesticating cattle, while llamas and alpacas were domesticated in South America.

Archaeologists consider the hunter-gatherer way of life as the original leisure time society. A few hours of foraging a day, combined with a hunt every few weeks, provided the necessities. If you survived early life when mortality was high, the modal or most common ages of death did not vary much from today's. For modern hunter-gatherer populations, the commonest age of death for those over age 15 is in the range of 68–78 years, which is not very different from the US (85 years) [51]. Your work depended on where you lived. Inuit people, Alaska Natives, mostly hunted and did not do much foraging, as few plants grew in the very far north. As agriculture spread, however, more work was needed to prepare soil, weed, irrigate, and harvest the crops. To increase the labor force, women had to produce more children, and their status subsequently declined.

Besides demanding more work, agriculture created a surplus of food, which led to greater social stratification as hierarchies and patriarchies emerged [52]. Moreover, in order to maintain crops, populations settled and became less mobile. As humans roamed less freely, they lived more closely together, enabling infectious diseases to spread. Crops became vulnerable to pests and famine, making periods of nutritional stress more common. Fields irrigated with rudimentary forms of surface water brought vector diseases such as malaria. And the work itself caused severe bone and joint stress, as crops were planted, weeded, and harvested – primarily by women – by bending over for long periods. Living in more enclosed settings meant cooking over open fires inside huts with minimal air circulation, causing severe respiratory illnesses. Health thus declined with the so-called progress of agriculture. Human skeletons became shorter as nutrition became less adequate. Signs of infectious and nutritional diseases appeared on bony remains, and there were more signs of trauma to the bones [53].

People lived more closely to their domesticated animals, facilitating infectious disease transmission from these animals to humans. Smallpox came from bovines, influenza from domesticated fowl, and eventually HIV/AIDS from nonhuman primates.

Fertility, the number of babies women birthed, increased in these agrarian societies to provide needed workers. Women no longer breastfed for long since they had to work in the fields, and there were more readily available weaning foods. As fertility increased, so did maternal mortality, as birthing was hazardous.

As hierarchies developed, feudalism emerged, and subsistence economies became more vulnerable to instability. Someone who owned land could take advantage of someone who lacked land, and therefore their own crops, by compelling them to labor in the fields in exchange for a portion of the harvest. By controlling the store of food and the land on which it was grown, these feudal lords could compel the poor not only to labor in the fields, but also to construct housing for their feudal lords and fortresses to protect them, and could also send the poor to war on their behalf.

Along with the rise in agriculture and increase in populations came the destruction of natural habitats. Our recent scourge with SARS-CoV-2 resulted from wild habitat loss and increasing contact with species, such as bats, that may harbor the virus.

This decline in health that came with the rise of agriculture continued for several thousand years, along with a rise in inequality and warfare. It wasn't until the last few hundred years that human health improved, with advances in sanitation, better standards of living, the discovery of antibiotics and vaccines, and other medical innovations.

A broad overview of the pathways to health and illness from prehistory to the present explores human origins, then the rise of agriculture, followed by the attendant impacts of colonialism leading to the health or mortality stratification seen globally today [54].

But even these innovations have their limits. For example, while the discovery of antibiotics, which treat bacterial infections, are heralded as advances, the beneficial evidence is limited. Consider tuberculosis (TB), which commonly affects the lungs. When deaths from lung TB were monitored in Minnesota from 1890 to 1975, there was a striking rise in rates of the disease until 1915, when TB sanitoria were opened. Then the number of deaths plummeted. By the time antibiotic treatment became available in 1949, the TB death rate was at only a fifth of its peak. Isolating those infected and providing good housing and food made a profound difference in death rates. Standards of living improved as well. While drug treatment of TB made a difference, it was not the key player in decreasing TB mortality [55]. Despite the availability of antibiotics and major improvements in TB treatment today, it remains the leading cause of death globally from infectious disease.

Similarly for vaccines. Take measles as an example. Church parish records in England kept birth and death records for centuries together with a "visual autopsy" diagnosis upon demise. Measles is easy to diagnose with its characteristic rash. The death rate for childhood measles remained very high until around 1900, when it plummeted. A vaccine wasn't available until 1968, by which time measles was a rare cause of death. Again, improved standards of living made a huge difference [56]. Today measles is resurging, however, linked to political and economic turmoil, as vaccines have become so politicized that they are no longer valued as the public health advance they once were. As a public health instructor and practitioner, I do not subscribe to the anti-vax movement which is a part of today's global tumult.

So what should a population do to be healthy? If we aren't that much healthier than our prehistorical ancestors, and the medical advances we've made aren't having a significant impact on our health, what should we do? Just tell the population to do what individuals do for their own health? Not exactly. There are many factors that affect population health that are more important than the aggregate of what individuals do. If we get these elements right, then perhaps what individuals do for their health is not that important, as was seen for TB and measles.

Consider Japan, the country with the longest-lived people in the world, where three times as many men smoke per capita as in the United States. Regard this as Japan's smoking paradox. The Japanese are doing something at the population level that allows a health-reducing personal behavior such as cigarette smoking to not harm their health as much as it would if they were in the United States. Contemplating Japanese men smoking so much and it having less adverse health impacts is challenging for most of us. That leads us to consider what makes a population healthy.

POPULATION HEALTH PERSPECTIVE

The Centers for Disease Control and Prevention (CDC, a branch of the United States Department of Health and Human Services) considers population health "as an interdisciplinary, customizable approach that allows health departments to connect practice to policy for change to happen locally." This vague approach can mean almost anything.

Here, I will consider population health as the health outcomes of groups of individuals and the distribution of such outcomes within that group. So what are they?

As Japan's smoking paradox illustrates, personal behaviors, although important, are not as important as we think. One can similarly address other individual health-related behaviors, such as exercise and diet. Yes, all of them matter a bit. But add all the parts together and it isn't enough to explain the range of health outcomes among nations.

At the beginning of this chapter it was pointed out that early life should be considered important, noting that the United States stands with Papua New Guinea as the only two countries worldwide not offering parents time and resources to care for their newborns. This is one example of a national population health policy applicable to the early years.

What else to consider? Public health now discusses the social determinants of health (SDOH). How should we define these social determinants? In the United States, Hawai'i is the healthiest state, in having the highest life expectancy of US states. Its Department of Health produced a 2011 report on social determinants. Its key graphic, Figure 3.1, shows a common Hawaiian geographic feature, namely a mountainside with a pass labelled *Mauka* (meaning toward the mountain), or upstream "root causes," followed by a cascade of factors impacting health [57]. At the bottom, *Makai* (meaning toward the water) are downstream effects in the ocean. In between is a big waterfall near the top and then a river emanating from the cataract to the ocean. In the ocean are downstream effects, namely all the chronic diseases we suffer from as we age. On one shore lay the usual risk factors we consider unhealthy: smoking, physical inactivity, and obesity. On the other shore is healthcare. Hawai'i puts these downstream. In the middle, where the water cascades downward, are the SDOH. They include racism, poverty, education, crime, and pollution. Above are the two critical elements: social/economic conditions and, above that, political context and governance. Hawai'i recognizes the importance of politics in our health. This view makes politics, the political choices we make, the most important determinants of health according to the health department of our healthiest state. Rather than being limited by the term SDOH then, we should speak of the broader determinants of health which include the more important political dimension.

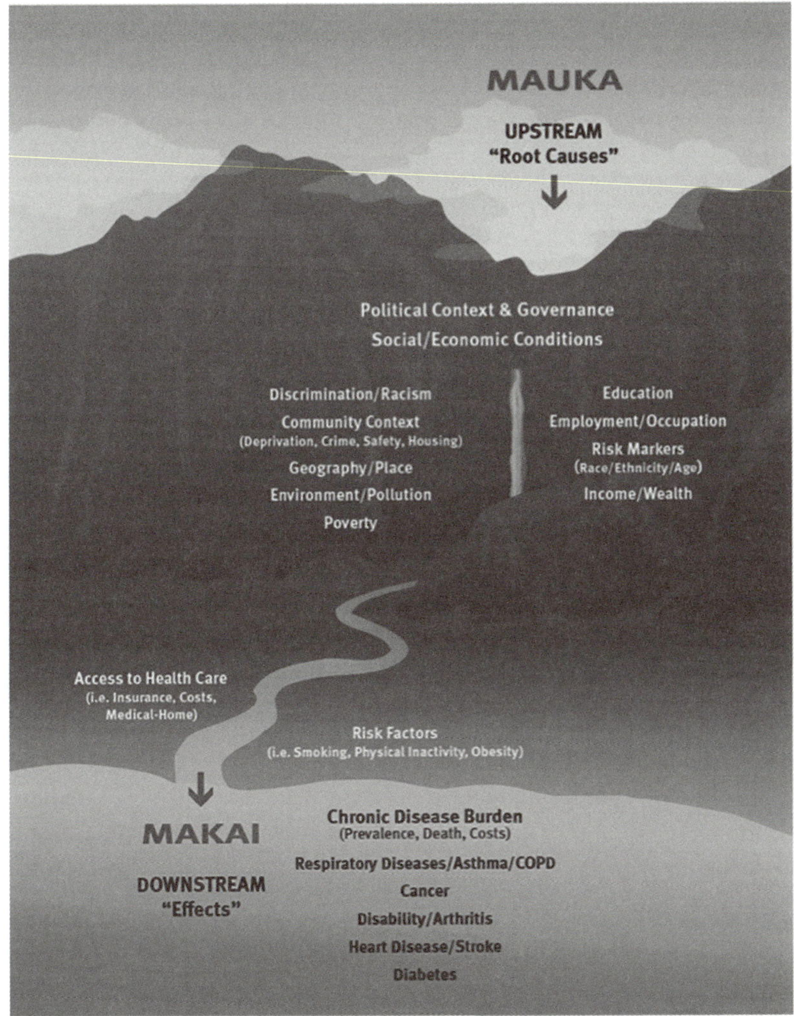

3.1 Determinants of health, from the Hawai'i State Department of Health [57]

Most people don't consider politics as the major issue to be addressed to produce health, despite what the Hawai'i State Department of Health says. Researchers at the Boston University School of Public Health carried out internet surveys of what matters for good health among the public in eight countries, including the United States. People were asked to rank the following in order of importance for healthy outcomes: built environment, childhood conditions, culture, education, employment conditions, genetics, healthcare, income and wealth, politics, and social support [32]. Americans ranked healthcare as most important and politics as last!

Defining politics is itself a political act. John Dewey said, "Politics is the shadow cast on society by big business," while Yanis Varoufakis, a former Greek finance minister, said, "Politics is about who has the right to tell whom what to do." Another is, "Who gets what, when and how?" [58]. An anthropological definition of politics is the control over resources and a political system is the system of mechanisms by which a social group organizes and controls power over resources. Let us consider politics as activities associated with the governance of a country or other jurisdiction, especially the debate or conflict among individuals or parties having or hoping to achieve power.

Power, a property of a population, represents the ability to cause pain or pleasure in others at little or no cost to yourself. Openly carrying a loaded gun is a way an individual expresses power in the US. The capacity to destroy the Earth through nuclear annihilation is how a nation expresses power. However it is deployed, being exposed to unfair power is stressful, which affects our health. Consider population health then as the recognition of, and collective reflection on, political power.

Big business has become the major political player in America, and increasingly around the world. Its power has led to a huge gap between rich and poor, especially in the United States. What impact does the gap in incomes or wealth in a country have on the health of its population? Economic inequality is an upstream factor, consistent with the graphic from the Hawai'i State Department of Health showcasing political context and governance.

Studies in 1979 began to link measures of income inequality among nations to their mortality measures. Hundreds of similar studies demonstrate that such inequality is associated with many bad health outcomes. The association is causal. More inequality produces worse health [59]. A population has inequality while an individual doesn't. Inequality is a collective relationship, and thus doesn't exist except in regard to an individual's connections within their society.

The relationship between health and inequality becomes apparent when we examine what occurs between mortality and income inequality in rich countries. And as I'll show in Chapter 5, it's a link also found at the US state level, and in other rich countries.

Different mortality outcomes within rich nations have been termed health inequities, health inequalities, and health disparities. The last term is in common use in the United States, where disparity just means a difference. The terms inequality and inequity refer to differences that are unjust or are both unjust and can be remedied. Consider the graphic analogy in Figure 3.2.

Three people of different heights at an athletic event stand behind a fence limiting their vision. If they each stand on a box of the same height, the tallest person gets the best view of the game, the second tallest can see the playing field while the shortest has their view obscured by the fence. This is equality, as they are all standing on the same size box. If the box from the tallest is given to the shortest, however, they all have the same view. This is equity. With equality, everyone has the same foundation, but with equity, everyone has the same outcome.

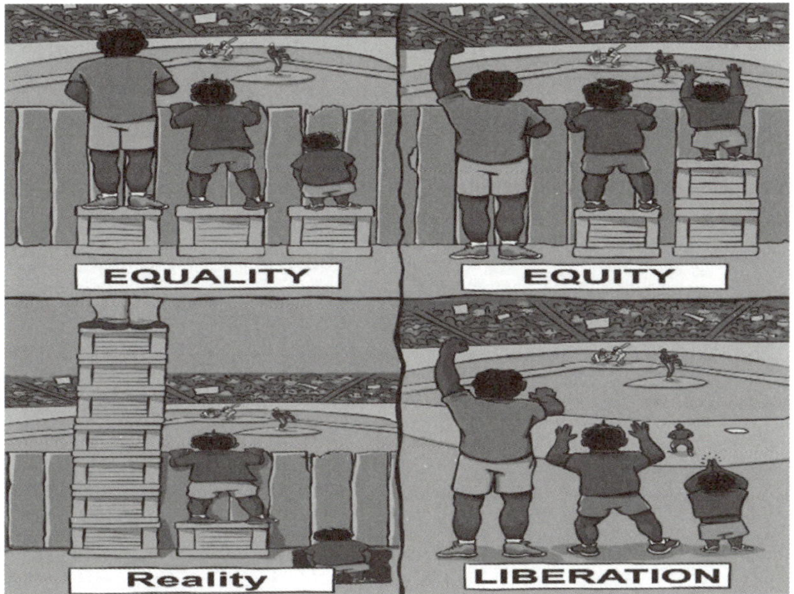

3.2 Equality and equity distinction
Image Credit: A collaboration between Center for Story-based Strategy (https://www.storybasedstrategy.org/the4thbox) and Interaction Institute for Social Change http://interactioninstitute.org/

One variation labelled *reality* has half a dozen boxes under the tall person while the short individual has to stand in a hole that puts their head at ground level. Another version removes the fence and is called *justice* or *liberation*, indicating that the cause of the inequity was addressed. One can expand this concept to look at those with physical and other disabilities. Impoverishment is lacking in these depictions. Poverty is avoidable insufficiency and is a policy choice. Why do those three people have to stand behind the fence? Why don't they have admission tickets to sit in regular seats as others do? Inequality is about unwarranted hierarchy; they shouldn't have to watch outside the spectator stands. However, it really is an *inequity*. Give them tickets to the stadium's event! Or, support all sports as a common good through taxing the rich, and don't charge for tickets at all!

How does inequality impact health? Consider a range of explanations [60] grouped into three realms.

The first realm relates to the curvilinear relationship between income and health. People with more income have better health than those with less. Poorer people have poorer health. The more income, the better the health. But as income increases into the high ranges, the health gains diminish. For someone making half a million dollars a year, an additional $10,000 of income will hardly improve that person's health, if at all. But increasing the income of a person making $25,000 by another $10,000 will have a sizable health benefit. Health gains thus diminish with greater incomes. So if you take a small chunk of income from the high earner and add it to the low earner, you will likely not impact the health of the high earner, but you will make a significant improvement in the health of the low earner. Average health thus improves when one takes a little – in the form of taxation – from the extremely rich and gives it to those more disadvantaged. Another interpretation is that inequality damages the health of the poor more than it impacts the health of the rich. The shape of the income health curve illustrates only a small part of the impact of income inequality on health.

Consider survival on the Titanic. When the Titanic sank in 1912, 60% of those holding first-class tickets survived, as did 40% of those with second-class tickets [61]. Among the crew and third-class passengers, however, only a quarter made it out alive. This socioeconomic gradient, poorer people having poorer outcomes, is found almost everywhere.

The second explanation, the psychosocial one, refers to the social comparisons we make. Income inequality changes how we behave with one another. An example used by Ichiro Kawachi describes the impact of air rage. Air rage is increasing on passenger airplanes: belligerent behaviors, drunken arguments, sexual advances and even assaults, and noncompliance with safety regulations. Jets with first-class seating have more air rage than those without [62,63]. Front boarding through the first-class cabin increases air rage among the first-class passengers more than when passengers board behind first class, as in jumbo jets. Seeing a divide between first or business class and cabin class rankles all of us, including those in first class. We similarly see road rage and other forms of aggressive behavior based on status. Those driving expensive cars and large SUVs are more likely to cut off other cars and even pedestrians, drive faster, and cause other havoc [64].

People around the world now exhibit more violent behaviors. These include mass shootings in the United States, various gender-based attacks in many countries, and other forms of violent conflict, often surrounding elections and other aspects of political processes. These behaviors can be ascribed to many factors, including the breakdown in rule of law, corruption of state institutions, increasing economic inequality, and resource scarcity exacerbated by the climate crisis, austerity, and wars – made all the more stressful as the threat of nuclear war looms. Social media not only facilitates the instantaneous and worldwide spread of information that provokes a sense of righteous rage (as we saw in the storming of the United States Capitol on January 6, 2021), but also makes it much easier to see what others have that we do not have, contributing to rage.

People who rank lower in a society's hierarchy may find opportunities where their status gives them privileges not found in their usual environment. One example comes from the United States' invasion of Iraq in 2003. Some US soldiers, who were mostly from lower socioeconomic circumstances – the so-called poverty draft – found themselves in positions of considerable authority inside prisons such as Abu Ghraib near Baghdad. Horrific pictures of torture and humiliation that US soldiers had carried out on Iraqi prisoners were leaked. Gloating smiles of the American enlisted men and women demonstrated how much they enjoyed exercising considerable power over their captives. These acts constituted war crimes. What about outside of wars?

When I was in medical school at Stanford in the early 1970s, the Stanford prison experiment took place. A group of students were jailers and another group prisoners in a simulated jail. The experiment had to be stopped after a week, however, because the student jailers began carrying out atrocities on their fellow-student prisoners. Both examples illustrate how being given roles in a hierarchical environment leads those with more power to torment others with less. Much more about such behaviors can be discussed [65].

Consider experiments with animals who reject being treated unequally. Primatologist Frans de Waal describes one with monkeys that can be found on YouTube.[1] Monkeys in cages are given a task and are rewarded on completion of the task, for example, by being given a piece of cucumber to eat. When monkeys see each other doing the same task and given the same reward, they are all satisfied. But if one monkey is given a grape the next time she completes the task, the other monkeys become outraged and rattle the cage bars. Studies with birds, dogs, and other animals show that these creatures prefer being treated fairly [66]. The stress of such inequality is a major pathway affecting health outcomes.

The third mechanism shows how the rich game the system to their further advantage. They already send their children to private schools, use legacy means to get them admitted to prestigious universities, live in gated communities, pay for enhanced security, and have concierge doctors at their beck and call. They have chauffeurs and private jets. They escape to island vacation paradises. And to avoid sharing their wealth through taxation, many shelter their income and wealth in offshore havens. Whatever tax they do pay is at a much lower percentage than the rest of us [67]. As they effectively pull away from society, we all lose social cohesion, namely the cooperation among us that benefits us all. Social capital can be defined as the resources that are accessed by individuals as a result of their membership of a network or a group. It encompasses features of social organization, such as trust, communication, and value generated by people working together [68].

During the COVID-19 era, it became apparent how the rich seceded from society, such as retreating on private planes to their third or fourth

---

[1] www.youtube.com/watch?v=lKhAd0TynyO.

home on a vacation island paradise to escape infection. They did not face income loss and actually profited from the pandemic. The poor, and those without college degrees, were more likely to be laid off than the rich or those with college degrees. They were also more likely to be exposed to the virus through their work, such as delivering food and groceries. Prices rose much more than wages, resulting in increasing profits and inflation, and opportunities to prosper from certain stocks affected by the pandemic disproportionately benefited the rich. As a result, the rich saw their wealth double in only a couple of years, while those living on the margins were bankrupted, lost their homes, or suffered other economic setbacks they've been unable to recover from. Yet the real price paid is that the US has the largest number of deaths from COVID-19 of any country [69]. As the time of writing, in early 2025, about 1 in 300 Americans has died from COVID-19.

Recall the root causes in the graphic from the Hawai'i State Department of Health: socioeconomic conditions and, above that, political context and governance. That image highlights the gap between richer and poorer. Let's call this political system that takes from the poor and gives to the rich a wealth pump.

HEALTH PROMOTION

Public health workers speak of health promotion. The 1986 Ottawa Charter defined health promotion as, "the process of enabling people to increase control over, and to improve, their health." The WHO takes a broader perspective, with its charter describing basic *prerequisites for health* which include peace, shelter, education, food, income, a stable ecosystem, sustainable resources, social justice, and equity. The WHO goes on to say that health promotion is based on a commitment to improving health and well-being through five pillars of action: building healthy public policy, creating supportive environments, strengthening community action, developing personal skills, and reorienting health (care) services. I added care to make the distinction advocated throughout this book.

Health promotion is thus much more than what individuals do to be healthy. It's about what our policy makers and national leaders can do to make us healthy.

GENDER AND HEALTH

In almost all countries today, women live longer than men. They have better survival for most diseases. The gender difference in life expectancy in rich nations today varies from a low of 4 years in the Netherlands and Israel to over 10 years in some former Soviet Union countries. The United States gap ranged from 6 to 7 years over the last 25 years of the last century and has dropped to around 5 years now.

The reasons for this difference are debatable. The suggested survival advantage has biological underpinnings: testosterone compromising male health, perhaps through more aggressive behaviors, the possible protective effect of menopause, and differences in inflammatory responses. One could say that men have an X chromosome deficiency disorder. The Y-chromosome has few genes. If an X is deficient in some way, women have another to draw on to enhance survival. We can thus consider women's health as superior to that of men.

Being a woman has big survival differences among countries related to many issues, including income inequality, gross domestic product, alcohol and tobacco consumption, socioeconomic adversity, and the nature of social relationships. In the United States, income inequality is especially important for limiting women's biological survival advantages [70,71].

By contrast, due to their almost universal second-class citizenship, the costs of patriarchal violence and exploitation, and the hazards of the gendered labor they are exposed to, women may have worse health throughout life, reporting more physical limitations, greater disability, and more cases of degenerative arthritis, among many conditions. But there is no doubt that women live longer than men.

GEOGRAPHY AND HEALTH

Regardless of your gender or the sex you are assigned at birth, where you live also matters for how long and how well you live. Consider the map in Figure 3.3 of US county life expectancy in 2019.

We find a 20-year life expectancy range among counties, with the darkest gray depicting the lowest life expectancy and the lightest gray

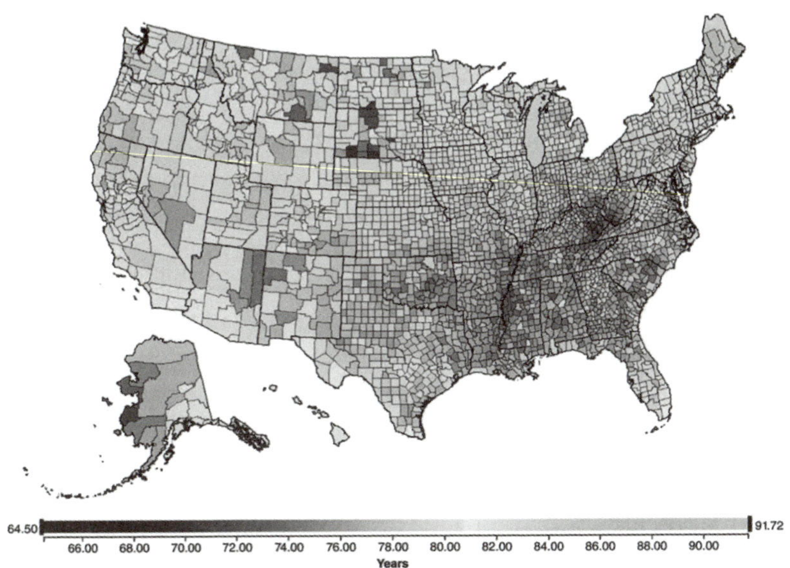

3.3 Life expectancy, US counties 2019 [72]

the highest. The darker tones are concentrated in the extended Mississippi River valley, together with Appalachia and the Southeast, with scatterings elsewhere. We see vast health inequities throughout the United States, with the worst outcomes found in Native American reservations in the upper Midwest. The best rates are found west of Denver in Colorado. These depictions can be refined for race, gender, economic status, and age, as well as for smaller units down to census tracts. They can map trends over time and disease frequencies as well as differing biological parameters.

Our World in Data is an extensive source of internet presentations with specific data sources, using an interactive format incorporating trend features that appeals to many media outlets.

Does geography determine your health destiny or is it something else? Can you move somewhere to be healthier? These questions are discussed in Chapter 9. Moving from sicker counties or states to healthier ones within the US while quite young, certainly before attaining the teenage years, may provide some health benefits.

More important are the social and economic conditions as well as political context and governance, as depicted by the Hawai'i State Department of Health. Rather than focus on smaller areas, we need to implement policies to make the entire nation healthier.

CULTURE AND HEALTH

Culture impacts the health of a society. Culture is difficult to define, and its population health impacts have not been subject to much rigorous study. Let's try to explain culture and then relate health outcomes to this phenomenon.

A common definition of culture is, "the language and accumulated knowledge, beliefs, practices, assumptions, and values that are passed between individuals, groups, and generations." There are hundreds of different definitions in the literature. Consider culture as "software of the mind" – as the "collective programming of the mind that distinguishes the members of one group or category of people from another" [73].

Geert Hofstede studied the values of employees of the International Business Machines Corporation (IBM) from 1967 to 1973. He categorized four dimensions to analyze cultural values. These were individualism–collectivism, uncertainty avoidance, power distance, and masculinity–femininity. Subsequent research in Hong Kong added long-term versus short-term orientation. Finally, he considered a sixth dimension, indulgence versus restraint. These could be quantified to give national scores and allow comparisons.

Richard Eckersley of the Australian National University studies the role of culture in determining health outcomes [74]. He argues that health production requires a complex systems analysis. Income inequality is only one factor in that system. In accepting the Hawai'i graphic shown earlier, political context and governance is a root cause, but also part of a complex system. But so is culture, which is not depicted in the graphic.

Consider Japan, with its stellar health outcomes and the much greater proportion of men who smoke cigarettes. Could culture be an explanatory factor? Their concept of *wa* or social harmony, typified by the observation that Japanese people do things together while Americans are much more likely to be alone in their pursuits, is an explanatory factor. Having social support alleviates stress and provides safeguards when you do become sick. You have people to care for you, and help you to get the attention you need. Other cultural factors could include diet (the Japanese eat small portions of fresh food, with red meat as an accent, rather than a main dish) and exercise (which is incorporated in daily lifestyles in Japan). It also helps that Japan has lower levels of inequality than many other developed countries.

RACISM AND HEALTH

The greatest burden of excess morbidity and mortality in the US, no matter what the measure of health, is inflicted upon Native Americans. Forced extermination of this population began with the arrival of European settlers over 500 years ago. The legacies of this violent conquest continue into the twenty-first century, with Native Americans who live on reservations having the worst health in the nation.

African Americans, as descendants of enslaved people, bear their own history and burden of excess morbidity and mortality. Fundamental cause theory explains outcomes. Economic and social disenfranchisement, as presented above, certainly qualifies. The household wealth of Black people is near zero while that of White people is closer to $200,000. Racism is the ideology underlying, upholding, and justifying interpersonal, institutional, and political discrimination, injustice, and violence. Racism intersects with resulting economic exploitation, social marginalization, and political disenfranchisement, which together are the fundamental causes of racial and ethnic health disparities [75].

Racism is perpetrated interpersonally, institutionally, and systemically in all American institutions, including whenever and wherever medical care is provided. When seeking medical care in the US, a Black person experiences more barriers and delays, worse treatments, more outright harm, and more negative outcomes than a White person, due to institutional racism. African Americans are less likely to receive pain medicine. They will receive fewer tests and investigations than White people, and their health outcomes and survival rates are worse [76]. Yet the reasons for these patterns of inequity go far beyond medical care.

Consider racism as the weaponization of difference for the purpose of exploiting, plus power to inflict this institutionally. Power structures opportunity (e.g. education, housing, safety, respect, votes, jobs, justice) and assigns value (worthy or unworthy, full of potential or full of menace) based on the social interpretation of how one looks. The range of responses to human visual difference and uses of human visual difference as hierarchy is called "racialization," though there is no biological foundation to the concept of race, which originated in the eighteenth century with the rise of colonial conquest.

While race has no biological foundation, there is a social reality to how we perceive different phenotypes (how our physical traits appear). Racism – ideologies of group inferiority and superiority that support discrimination and domination of groups of people based on their phenotype – has been used as a way to subordinate different groups based mostly on myths about genetic or biological predispositions. Through the implementation of destructive policies such as segregation and redlining, which restrict resources to individuals and communities, racism affects where people live, the quality of education they receive, what job opportunities they have, how much they are paid, and other economic factors that affect health and healthcare. Racism also affects how healthcare providers perceive and respond to patient concerns. All these manifestations of racism have real biological implications by negatively affecting healthcare access and health outcomes. The connection between racism and exposure to economic immiseration and social stress, and the influence of both on health, thus become very clear.

Besides higher mortality rates, and dying earlier than other groups, Native Americans and African Americans experience higher rates of excess morbidity, illness, and disease that would not occur if they were not living in a racist society: lower birthweight, more preterm deliveries, diabetes, hypertension, and many more adverse health outcomes, including worse dental health. There is more asthma (and worse outcomes for those who have asthma) among Native and Black Americans than among White Americans. Native and Black people and Pacific Islanders with kidney disease requiring dialysis are less likely to be recommended for a kidney transplant (a better way to control renal failure) than White people. We see this intentional burden of death and disease continuing across generations, from Africans who were trafficked and enslaved to their descendants in the present in the United States. This ongoing suffering has been called posttraumatic slave syndrome [77]. There are few medical data about the millions of Black people who were enslaved in the US during the transatlantic slave trade and up to the Civil War, but it is likely that most did not have good health in that era. We do know that, in the era of enslaving people in the United States, at one year of age, enslaved babies were small [78]. Enslavers asserted that the human beings they enslaved had high pain thresholds, and operated on them without any anesthesia, forming the roots of medical experimentation on and torture of Black people that continued in cases such as the Tuskegee Syphilis Study [79].

Low birthweight is more frequent among US-born Black people than among non-US-born Black and US-born White people [80]. Yet after some years living in the US, those differences start to wane, and the next generations of descendants of Black immigrants soon have high rates of low birthweight and other negative maternal/infant outcomes similar to those of US-born Black families. This suggests that racial/ethnic disparities in low birthweight are most likely associated with social determinants than with other possible causes. For example, the more racist the policies at the state level, the higher are both Black and White mortality rates. One explanation is that this pattern results from cuts in social service expenditures or the refusal of federal social safety net funds in former slave-owning, -trafficking, and -breeding states. The worst outcomes for White people tend to be where they are the worst for Black and Latinx people: the Mississippi Delta and the Mexican borderlands. Welfare and social expenditures in these regions are the lowest in the nation, so the institutional violence harms all marginalized communities [81].

WHAT DIET IS BEST FOR HEALTH?

One feature of culture that is considered central to health is diet. Let's consider this factor more closely. There's no shortage of dietary advice. Eat this, avoid that. The Mediterranean diet will change your life. A vegan diet will lengthen your life. What can be deduced from this plethora of recommendations? To study seriously the impact of diet on health would require a long-term cohort study in which different groups of people would consume different standardized diets over a lifetime to gauge their impact. Such research is impossible to carry out. A review paper [82] considering existing knowledge on this subject concluded that "the weight of evidence strongly supports a theme of healthful eating while allowing for variations on that theme. A diet of minimally processed foods close to nature, predominantly plants, is decisively associated with health promotion and disease prevention and is consistent with the salient components of seemingly distinct dietary approaches."

In medical school one nutritionist advised us to eat local foods that spoil but eat them before they do. Given all the different diets Americans eat and the fact that none of us can claim stellar health, what dietary advice can I offer? Eat a wide variety of foods, eat those you enjoy that are more plant based, and don't eat too much of them. Avoid highly and ultra-processed foods which are heavily marketed and can be addictive.

In the Hawai'i State Department of Health mountainside graphic on the determinants of health earlier in Chapter 3, diet is not listed but could have been included as one of the risk factors, along with obesity and physical activity, that was as far downstream as could be and not be in the ocean. Much more important to your health, however, is having access to basic resources. Recall that political context matters most. With a huge, mostly unregulated food industry whose profits are produced by getting us to eat more processed foods, this is a huge challenge that is intensified by the burgeoning promotion of drugs for weight loss.

Limiting exposure to certain possible harmful chemicals in foods is challenging in modern society. Some, such as trans-fats, were a common part of the diet but strong efforts were made to remove them. Some would put refined sugar in this category. We consume huge amounts of sugar these days, which is added to most highly processed foods. Like processed foods, trying to limit sugar-sweetened drinks is difficult because of strong industry pressure to consume them.

While eating a healthy plant-based diet is important, trying to find the optimal diet to be healthy is a distraction from working on population-level factors that produce health. So if diet isn't the most important factor in determining our health, what about the environment? Could environmental exposures be more important than diet?

PHYSICAL AND CHEMICAL ENVIRONMENTAL HAZARDS

Many worry about the health risk attributed to physical or chemical environmental hazards. We hear many reports about exposure to this or that toxin in our food supply, water, or air that causes cancer, respiratory disorders, or other health problems. How hazardous are these risks we hear about all the time? Studying environmental hazards is problematic. High levels of exposure to a harmful substance over a short time can produce serious toxicities. From 1932 to 1968, people in Minamata Bay, Japan, were exposed to high levels of methylmercury in contaminated fish and shellfish when mercury oxide was discharged by a factory owned by the Chisso Corporation. Victims suffered from a chronic neurological disease (now called Minamata disease), with the first report of a patient in 1956. It took a long time before the connections were made and the source of the toxicity was eliminated. There were 2,265 victims, with 1,784 deaths and many more born with serious birth defects. Despite knowing of these serious health impacts, however, it wasn't until 2004 that the company began to clean up the area.

Lessons from this disaster are that exposure to environmental toxins can be insidious. Even with high exposure it may take years to recognize the damage. But what about the health impacts of lower levels of exposure, often over long time periods? The answers are speculative at best. But in the past 75 years we have learned that exposure over a critical part of the life cycle, especially during pregnancy, can produce disastrous outcomes. Yet people, families, communities, and nations vary in their attempts to limit these exposures. Consider the following examples.

Exposure to lead, a heavy metal, leads to many health issues and has been described since the second century BCE. Low levels of lead exposure in children causes developmental brain damage. But as late as 1982 the lead industry denied this health risk. Gasoline used to be refined with lead, but this practice has been stopped in most (but not all) parts of the world. Lead was added to paints until this practice was banned in 1978. Millions of American homes still have leaded paint in them that can result in toxic exposure, especially with the danger of eating paint chips, especially for impoverished, young children living in unregulated, old-stock housing. Perhaps half of US children under age six have detectable levels of lead in their blood [83]. This decreases learning abilities and compromises educational outcomes. Such soft signs or outcomes can easily be missed or not attributed to lead exposure. Lead exposure related to paint is most common in older buildings and homes that have been poorly maintained, so people with no access to adequate income, particularly people of color and immigrants, who are often forced to live in segregated areas not protected by residential zoning laws, are more likely to be exposed to lead paint. A common form of exposure comes from old casement windows, which release fine particles of leaded paint dust each time they are opened or closed.

Thalidomide, touted as a sedative without side effects, was a drug commonly used in Europe in the late 1950s and early 1960s for nausea and vomiting during pregnancy, as well as many other conditions. Exposure led to a number of serious congenital disorders. Although the US Food and Drug Administration (FDA) had officially kept thalidomide off the market, Merrell, an American pharmaceutical corporation, provided samples to doctors to hand out to patients. Many babies were born with congenital disabilities, but their mothers were never told that they had received thalidomide [84]. In contrast, thalidomide was legally used in Canada and many other countries, so those children received some support for their lifelong disabilities. Thalidomide is a pharmaceutical that can be valuable to some, for example for treating leprosy complications and multiple myeloma, but its use must be carefully restricted.

It is difficult to isolate the impact of chemicals to which everyone is exposed, and the limitless combination of chemicals to which we are exposed further complicates our understanding of their health impacts. We are continuously and increasingly exposed to many potential environmental substances. In this country, attempts are made to remove a substance produced by industry only after it is found to be hazardous. In Europe the precautionary principle is more often considered, namely when the impacts of a substance are unknown or possibly harmful, we should err on the side of caution, so the substance should not be used or manufactured.

People who are impoverished, Black, Indigenous, and people of color (BIPOC) and other communities who are marginalized in various ways have more exposure to such hazards. Environmental justice draws attention to the threats of environmental racism. For example, there is evidence for global warming, such as CO_2 emissions, being impacted by income inequality. (In Chapter 5 we will look at the effects of particulate matter in our air.) We will later consider epigenetics as a biological tool to understand the role of the environment in this process[65,85].

We are exposed to per- and polyfluoroalkyl substances (PFAS) that were produced in the 1930s by researchers at DuPont looking for durable stable refrigerants. The properties of PFAS led to them having multiple industrial and consumer uses. They are considered forever chemicals, since in the natural world it takes thousands of years for them to break down. In many nonhuman animal studies, PFAS have been shown to be toxic. They are not safe in humans and especially hazardous among the youngest. They have also been linked to chronic diseases in adulthood. Yet they are found in numerous products including organic eggs, freshwater fish, and almost everywhere including Antarctic snow, and even in the human body where they are linked to proteins in our blood. With plastic chemicals and substances almost everywhere on the planet, all of us have them in our bodies, and they are almost impossible to avoid.

Are these ubiquitous chemicals, whose production is unregulated, hazardous to our health? Almost certainly [86]. Some PFAS molecules resemble fatty acids and so are incorporated into our cells. In the liver they probably contribute to nonalcoholic fatty liver disease. They are endocrine disruptors and likely obesogens (meaning they make us fat). It has been shown that PFAS cross the placenta and are excreted in breast milk. A large US study demonstrated that their presence contributes to lower birthweight [87]. This leads to many consequences, including metabolic syndrome. The brain may be the most affected organ.

Can we measure PFAS or plastic exposure in different populations or nations to better understand their causal effect on health? Not yet. Consider limiting exposure to them as another important environmental issue that will require a global response.

While it is easy to believe that the toxic environmental swamp we live in causes the poor health status of the United States, the argument can't be sustained at the population level. While living in an area where you are exposed to environmental toxins or hazards may jeopardize your health, Americans who have the financial resources to live or work far from the quagmire still have worse health than people in other nations living in less eco-friendly circumstances. Political circumstances matter, especially the way economic inequality affects our health. These health effects begin very early in life. In the next chapter, we'll explore how early life shapes the years that follow.

CHAPTER FOUR

Early Life Lasts a Lifetime

It is easier to build strong children than to repair broken men.

Frederick Douglass

As we go from the womb to the tomb, about half of our health as adults is programmed by conditions in the first 1,000 days after conception.

The fetus lives in a womb with a view, namely it gets signals from the mother about what the outside world is going to be like. Will it be nurturing and safe with necessary attention provided so that the period of fetal development in the uterus is sufficient for the organs to reach their full functioning potential? Or is it a hostile world, where once you are born, you must be on your guard to survive to reproduce? In such circumstances, maternal responses to stress can lead to early onset of labor and preterm birth. Many problems are associated with being born preterm and of low birthweight, a large number of which are associated with poverty and various conflicts that lead to low social status [88]. While there are many reasons a fetus may be born early, one big factor is maternal stress. Stress signals from the mother tell the body that it had better hurry up and give birth. So, you come out of the womb early, and have a low birthweight (less than 2,500 g or 5.5 pounds). Birthweight is the easiest measured indicator of how well a fetus developed *in utero*.

As with many health-related situations in this book, my statements refer to populations and not to individual circumstances. If you give birth to a low-birthweight baby, you should not blame yourself for the conditions that led to this, most of which are related to economic marginalization. The culprit is the society that produces the conditions that lead to such outcomes. We shall see later that stress in the US is among the highest levels in the world. This contributes to the chances of Americans having low-birthweight babies. Even so your child may do just fine.

At the same time, environmental factors acting in early life, up to about age two, impact human longevity. These processes, which begin in the womb or even sooner, explain the adult development of the many chronic diseases that afflict us as we age.

PRECONCEPTION: STRESS BEFORE THE FIRST NINE MONTHS

The effects of early-life situations on adult health begin before you are conceived. Severe stresses produce biological changes in the parent before conception that influence the fetus and, thereafter, the child. If the mother-to-be experiences a major life trauma, for example the death of her parent, child, or spouse, a divorce or separation from her partner, or fertility problems, without adequate support, she may be at an increased risk of giving birth to a low-birthweight infant. A higher risk does not mean a certainty. A study by researchers from the University of Wisconsin published in 2013 looked at American mothers in a birth cohort who bore children in 2001 [89]. They found that stressful life events, as listed above, prior to conception impacted birth outcomes. These included bodily processes that lead to negative birth outcomes, as well as coping mechanisms for stresses, for example smoking, that might contribute to low birthweight. They suggested that stress in the preconception period might be more important for birth outcomes than stress that occurs during pregnancy. Decreasing overall stress in US society might be extremely important for improving women's health and that of the next generation. A follow-up study with a different birth cohort by the same group looked beyond birthweight to examine toddler health when they were 9 and 24 months old to substantiate the importance of preconception stress on producing very-low-birthweight babies [90]. These kids already had health problems when examined at 9 and 24 months.

A subsequent Australian study pointed to preconception stress having more effect on low birthweight among firstborn babies. They also found that this effect was greater for female than for male babies [91]. We can expect outcomes of preconception stress to vary among nations for a variety of reasons. The United States has among the highest levels of stress of all nations, and considerably more than in Australia. A study from Pittsburgh looked at community violence, aggression between adults, and caregiving when the girls were growing up, and found links to low birthweight as well as slower fetal growth than expected when these girls later had babies [92]. As with pretty well every health condition, the burden is worse for African Americans [93]. Among the reasons are the intergenerational stressors and ongoing experiences of racial oppression since enslavement, discussed in the last chapter. A review of many studies suggests that childhood stress in the parent-to-be matters more for subsequent pregnancy outcomes than stress *just before* conceiving [94].

What about the father's stress before a child is conceived? If the American father has a chronic illness condition, it is more likely to lead to a stillbirth [95]. Stresses in the early life of the father, such as emotional neglect and abuse, physical neglect and abuse, and sexual abuse, have been associated with newborn brain changes [96]. An MRI scan can demonstrate specific newborn brain changes that may predispose that person to various health conditions. Long-term follow-up is required to understand the impact of paternal stress on the progeny.

In this section we have talked about parental stress impacting the unborn fetus even before it has been conceived. Many other factors have been implicated. Another perspective considers the zero trimester as the time before pregnancy begins in which conditions help explain the substandard US health status. This has led to prepregnancy or preconception healthcare promotion programs together with attendant advice to the mother-to-be. For example, women of reproductive age are being told by the Centers for Disease Control and Prevention (CDC) to eschew alcohol if not using birth control. Critics of this perspective suggest that women are not merely vessels for someone else. The focus here is to lay the blame on society, which involves all of us.

We conclude that something about living in the highly stressed United States before a baby is conceived impacts the health of both the parents and the fetus. Could that be an important reason why health in the US is not so good, and even declining? If preconception stress matters so much, it suggests that our health is not under our individual control. Let's consider what happens with and after conception.

THE FIRST NINE MONTHS

Birthweights range from around 2 to 10 pounds. The larger the birthweight, the more likely better fetal development occurs. David Barker first linked low birthweight to later heart attacks in a 1986 study with Clyde Osmond. They looked at infant mortality rates between 1921 and 1925 in regions of England and Wales and found strong associations with heart disease mortality from 1968 to 1978 [97]. They argued that living in conditions of impoverishment, with inadequate nutrition in early life, led to later heart attack deaths. Thus began the fetal origins of adult disease paradigm.

Barker wanted other sources to link low birthweight to adult health, and found good records of birth cohorts in Helsinki, Finland. There he discovered that slow fetal growth and slow growth during infancy followed by rapid catch-up growth leads to coronary heart disease, including heart attacks and type 2 diabetes [98]. Slow growth *in utero* makes the infant more vulnerable to the stress effects of low socioeconomic status and low income, and makes them more likely to develop coronary heart disease in adulthood.

Many studies validate that birthweight is a critical indicator of fetal development. If you were born with low birthweight, this does not doom you to poor adult health, however. It is just more likely you'll face health challenges, some of which may be alleviated by social support. One study looked at how birthweight might affect the brain and its development.

This study considered all births in Florida from 1992 to 2002 and matched birthweight with standardized test score outcomes in grades 3 to 8 for those attending public schools there [99]. The study of over 1.3 million births found that birthweight is associated with cognitive development as measured by these tests across a wide range of family socioeconomic statuses and ethnicities. There was an increasing monotonic (rising steadily) relationship between birthweight and test scores, peaking around 4,300 g or 9.5 pounds. The higher the birthweight, the higher the test score. When the mother's educational status was considered, the same monotonic relationship between birthweight and test scores was seen for the children of mothers who didn't complete high school, those who did but had no college education, those with some college education, and those who completed college. For mothers who did not graduate from high school and whose child was at the peak birthweight level, that child's test scores were comparable to the low-level test scores of the children whose mothers graduated from high school. Similarly, for mothers who had some college education, namely whose children were at the upper birthweight end, their children's test scores were comparable to those of children with low birthweights whose mothers were college graduates. When stratified by racially oppressed groups, birthweights and test scores were lower among children born to Black non-Latinx mothers and higher among those born to Asian non-Latinx mothers, consistently preserving the educational measure relationship with birthweight, namely the higher the birthweight the higher the scores on the standardized tests. The quality of the schools attended did not impact the results. For each birthweight, there was a wide range of possible educational outcomes, so a low-birthweight newborn might later do well on the tests. It was just less frequent.

This study, tracking over a million children, has important implications pointing out the effects of being born of low birthweight. Maternal education and the experience of anti-Black racial hierarchy are associated with birthweight, which, in turn, is associated with performance on standardized tests, used as a proxy for cognitive functioning. This assumes that cognitive function can be accurately measured by the standardized tests run by for-profit businesses, which are routinely administered to children in the United States. Interpretation of these data is greatly hampered by the lack of consideration of nutrition, household employment and income, and housing safety and security variables, all factors that mediate maternal health, fetal development, and birthweight, for which maternal education may be a proxy [100]. A vibrant literature regarding racial and social class being embedded in standardized testing that is carried out in the US adds further nuance and complexity to explaining these associations, and challenges simple conclusions. Nevertheless, the various categorizations of those born with low birthweight suggest an impact on brain development and cognitive function.

Some readers may consider this material to house elements of biological determinism that was voiced in the past and subsequently discredited, but still haunting today's social and medical sciences. Biology is inseparably intertwined with the environment in both local and global ways, so much so that whether talking about genes, brains, or anything in between, it no longer makes sense to ask, "What does this gene/neurotransmitter/brain do?"; instead, we should ask, "What does it do in a particular environment?" The function of the brain can never be understood outside the context of the body in which it is happening, nor outside the society in which the person in that body is living.

Research from Georgetown University looked at a birth cohort of twins and found that the impacts of low birthweight on cognitive and socio-emotional outcomes were stronger for children living in lower-income households [101]. In the United States public education continues to be our single most important engine for reducing inequality. Higher levels of education, however, do not eliminate people's exposure to the stressors of racial inequity and institutional violence [102]. This is exemplified by African American mothers who graduated from college suffering a greater risk of dying in childbirth than any other racialized group of that educational status, and a greater relative risk of dying in childbirth than their sisters with less education [103]. A college education does not protect them from the stressors of anti-Black racism. In fact, it may expose them to greater racial stressors as they face hostilities in institutions that were not designed for them to succeed, and where they may be racially and socially isolated and targeted. Let's consider how an element of biology might be involved.

The placenta, the interface between mother and fetus, nourishes the fetus and removes waste products. Characteristics of this organ, including its size and dimensions, relate to health issues such as having high blood pressure in adulthood. The placenta has to get oxygen and nutrients to the fetus.

Maternal stress can be transmitted to the fetus via stress hormones crossing the placenta. Stress hormones secreted by the mother trigger release of placental stress hormones that enter the fetal circulation, as well as having maternal stress-induced effects on the placenta. Maternal stress hormones may constrict blood flow to the placenta, thereby lowering oxygen and glucose delivery to the fetus, leading to health compromises. Recent research shows that long-term effects, such as heart disease, obesity, asthma, and several forms of cancer, may be influenced by the way the placenta grows. Ongoing maternal stress modifies how the placenta works in ways that can compromise fetal organ development, with adult health consequences [104].

In order to learn more about these complex physiological responses to stress, rather than take subjects and expose them to various stresses and observe the outcomes, something considered unethical today, we can look at certain stressful events that happened and create a natural experiment.

For example, the Dutch Hunger Winter, from November 1944 to May 1945 in the Netherlands, saw rations during World War II limited to less than 1,000 calories a day. Children born to women who were pregnant during this period were followed to adulthood. Those exposed to famine in the early period of gestation were more likely to have many bad health outcomes: mental disorders, altered cognitive function, altered blood coagulation, female obesity, heightened stress sensitivity, coronary artery disease, and breast cancer [27]. Those exposed in mid-gestation had kidney and lung diseases, as that was the period those organs were developing. Exposure throughout gestation led to glucose intolerance characteristic of type 2 diabetes. Worse health was found in those who were then born of women who themselves were born during this time. This represents an intergenerational transfer of compromised health.

This natural experiment considered nutritional stress in the womb, but other studies demonstrate the impact of other kinds of stress during pregnancy. Children born of pregnant women exposed to the psycho-social stress of the 2005 Hurricane Katrina in the US, as well as those affected by the 2001 collapse of the World Trade Center towers, have had subsequent health and developmental issues [105,106,107]. These include fetal deaths, preterm births, and lower birthweight. After the attack on the World Trade Center towers, a study found that Arab-named pregnant women in California had increased prevalence of low birthweight as well as preterm deliveries, leading researchers to consider the depth of fear and stress caused by anti-Muslim and anti-Arab discrimination, mistreatment, and violence [108]. The then US president named some countries the "axis of evil," which included Iran and Iraq, and implicated Arabs as the culprits. This led to discriminatory practices toward anyone perceived as being from the Middle East, including hate crimes. The 2016 presidential election increased the rate of preterm births in New York City and among US Latina and African American women due to heightened ethnic harassment [109]. Sociopolitical stressors of racism, anti-immigrant and misogynistic messages, and violence, strongly impacted the families of Black, Indigenous, and people of color (BIPOC) across the country, which, in turn, influenced the early life of those born into such a conflicted world.

Other important external environmental factors affect birth outcomes. For example, if a Black pregnant person witnesses or is otherwise exposed to a police killing of another Black person, they are more likely to go into stress-induced, early-onset labor, causing that infant to be born prematurely and, thus, making them more likely to be of low birthweight [110]. This extreme bystander harm caused by constant unsanctioned state violence is not additive, but multiplicative to the already heightened risks for negative birth outcomes African American people face.

Excess maternal stress during pregnancy has been shown to affect birth outcomes and the health of progeny in later life, manifesting as various diseases. Serious stressors include armed conflicts (wars) and other social determinants of health. While the rich wage most wars, it is mostly the poor who die [111,112].

Another way to consider why the first nine months *in utero* are so important to our health later in life is to look at cell division, a sensitive period easily impacted by several factors, including stress, but also pollution, radiation, drugs, and toxic chemicals, among many others. The ovum was made during your mother's fetal development in your maternal grandmother's womb. Thus, your grandmother's circumstances affect your health, a well-demonstrated finding. Once fertilized by your father's sperm, the ovum is called a zygote, which divides about 42 times to produce the full-term fetus. So many divisions in nine months is a short period for good things to happen, or to go wrong or to go badly. After being born, there are only 5 further cycles of cell division over almost 20 years to produce you. If we seriously want to impact individual- or population-level health outcomes, we should concentrate our efforts on the first nine months, rather than the ensuing two decades [113].

The country where you live matters. Consider the distribution of low birthweight among socioeconomic groups in the English-speaking countries Australia, Canada, the United Kingdom and the United States. The US has the highest rate of low birthweight, as well as the greatest socioeconomic inequality [100]. Something is not going right in America.

So, does it get any better after we're born?

STUDYING EARLY LIFE

Clyde Hertzman studied the 1958 British birth cohort (all those born in Britain during the first week of March 1958) [114]. He demonstrated that a few key markers of what happens to you between birth and age seven can affect your subsequent health as much as what happens afterwards [115]. These "latent effects" were birthweight, growth measured by height at age seven, social–emotional status at that age and parental interest in education. Based on these few markers, Hertzman sought to show that some individuals will have good outcomes, while others may not. This developmental origins of health and disease (DOHaD) paradigm provides a rich source of validated studies on early life. Conditions in early life can affect health for a lifetime.

UP TO AGE TWO (1,000 DAYS AFTER CONCEPTION)

Chapter 3 pointed out that human babies are born totally helpless and unable to care for themselves, requiring others, such as parents, to care for them over many years. Parenting varies tremendously around the world for cultural, historical, and political reasons. But one constant is breastfeeding, which has important advantages for later health [45]. In today's world, however, mothers may have to make many compromises to breastfeed.

John Bowlby, a British psychiatrist studying orphans in World War II, explored the concept of secure attachment of an infant to a mother-like figure that nourished the newborn. He considered the Western nuclear family context to understand early life. There followed the Bowlby–Ainsworth infant attachment model that a baby has a mother who is sensitive to her or his signals in the first year of life [116]. The child becomes capable of exploring its world knowing there is a secure base to return to. As the child grows up, the mother figure continues to be responsible for care. This concept, secure attachment, is bound in the model of the Western middle-class nuclear family, common in the middle of the twentieth century.

Such a colonial perspective did not consider the many ways infants and children are reared throughout the world. There may be several parental figures in the household, or nearby, who hold and nurse infants. They can provide skin-to-skin infant care during day and night with responsive feeding and co-sleeping. Alloparenting, or allomothering, is commonly found globally. *Allo* means not the self, but of the same species. Thus, alloparenting refers to communal care of the child, such as found throughout human evolution, and in some tribal and other societies today [117]. The core tenets of attachment theory are valid. The infant or child has to feel that they have a nurturing emotional relationship with one or more adults [118].

A natural experiment of zero parenting occurred in Romania when abortion was outlawed in the 1970s. One consequence of the abortion ban was that infants were regularly abandoned. The state collected these babies and housed them in orphanages that were inadequately staffed. Infants, toddlers, and children were left unattended, sometimes restrained in cribs. Humanitarian relief agencies discovered hundreds of thousands of such children in 1989. Even after they were adopted, follow-up studies demonstrated extreme mental and physical challenges that well-meaning parenting later could not change [119]. Similarly, adoption studies carried out in Chinese and Russian institutions, characterized as having psychosocial deprivation, also demonstrate development problems among children who were not held or provided with much physical contact or interaction as babies and toddlers [119]. Providing nurturing stimulation in early life is critical for good adult health outcomes.

US attachment issues are complex. As previously noted, the US is one of only two populous countries in the world that does not have a national policy granting paid maternity leave [49]. Most American mothers return to work shortly after having a baby. Lack of safety, as well as food and housing insecurity, make parenting here challenging. Single parenting is common. A variety of care arrangements need to be made that may not be ideal for the infant. Low rates of exclusive breastfeeding are common within the US, which have their own adverse health effects. Grandmothers used to do considerable allomothering, but as families splinter and increasingly live far apart, grandmothering is now less common. Changing family dynamics leave many American children having three or more primary caregivers in their early years. High rates of teen births also contribute, as there could be many teen parent figures who may not be prepared for parenting a newborn.

We are led to conclude that parenting during early life has much variation throughout the world and there is no one right way. The US situation may not be ideal for many children growing up here. There is a strong research base relating early-life attachment issues to later health, both mental and physical [120]. One example associates attachment style with the mortality rate from diabetes: there is a lower risk of death among those with secure attachment [121]. For those working in clinical psychology, mental healthcare and psychiatry, and for those who treat people's mental health problems, looking at a person's early-life issues helps the therapist gain an understanding of their mental health issues in adulthood.

CONDITIONS IN EARLY LIFE AND TRAUMA

Trauma, whether physical or psychological, plays a key role in early life. We learned just how significant early childhood trauma can be in the study of adverse childhood experiences (ACEs) that began in the 1970s. Dr. Vincent Felitti used supervised fasting to help control rising obesity in his patients at the Kaiser Permanente San Diego Medical Center. Under clinical conditions he was able to get some patients to lose 100 pounds in a year. Unexpectedly, many of these women would quickly put that weight back on. He discovered that these women had been sexually abused as children. As they lost so much weight, they would become attractive to men, triggering their abuse memories. Regaining the weight felt less of a hazard. Their weight was their "body armor."

Together with Dr. Robert Anda, Dr. Felitti then studied how common such childhood experiences were in the Kaiser Permanente population. They followed those enrolled in the clinic for many years to see what happened to adult health for those reporting abuse as children. They all had healthcare insurance. Their astounding results were published in 1998 [122]. More than half of the survey population had one or more ACEs out of a possible total of seven. Three of these ACEs are categories of abuse, including physical, emotional, and sexual. Then there is emotional and physical neglect. Finally, ACEs can include household dysfunction such as mental illness, having a close family member incarcerated, a mother treated violently, substance abuse among a close family member, and parental divorce. The more ACEs one had reported, the more adverse adult health behaviors they engaged in and the more adult diseases they suffered, including heart attacks, cancer, lung disease, skeletal fractures, and liver disease – all leading causes of death.

Those with higher ACE scores are more likely to be on antipsychotic drugs; to experience early sexual intercourse, teen pregnancy and paternity, and injection drug use; to attempt suicide; and to die early. The higher the ACE score, the greater the risk of dying. In fact, having 6 or more ACEs appeared to shorten one's life by some 20 years. Emotional abuse ACEs were more likely to lead to suicidal behaviors. The COVID-19 pandemic further increased the adverse impact of ACEs on mental health [123]. Subsequent studies demonstrated that having inadequate resources throughout childhood may expose people to more ACEs, but ACEs are reported by people from across the socioeconomic spectrum.

Vincent Felitti and Robert Anda observed that [124]:

> Clearly, much of what we see in adult medical practice and as current major public health problems has its origins in what was present but unrecognized in pediatrics. There is a need to move from our current symptom-responsive approach in primary care to the comprehensive approach that was conceived but not attained – a biopsychosocial approach.

Despite the fact that, as stated many times above, it is not individual behavior which accounts for most of our health outcomes, our healthcare approach in the US typically "blames the victim" and tries to change behaviors that are considered to lead to worse health. These so-called risk factor behaviors may be ways in which individuals cope with their early-life issues.

More broadly, ACEs can be considered to have three realms: those that happen within the family (the ACE study), those that happen in the community (substandard wages, jobs, poverty, violence, wars, racism), and those that are environmental (earthquakes, air pollution, global warming). But the domain used so far is mostly at the personal or family level.

The original ACE study's findings, published in 1998, have been widely circulated and led to the field of treating early-life trauma and its consequences. However, there are flaws in the way it has been used. The study itself asked subjects what their early-life experiences were when they were adults. The study did not assess the intensity or duration or chronicity of the abuse, nor the age at which it occurred. Thus, the ACEs score is a crude measure of childhood stress that should not be used as an individual standardized screening tool as, say, blood pressure is. If your blood pressure is significantly and chronically elevated, you will most likely be advised to have some intervention and subsequent monitoring. Your individual ACE score should not be used as such a screening tool. Nor should it be used to label certain populations as deficient and requiring intervention.

The study's results do not mean that one's personal experiences caused their adult health problems, although that is how it is often considered today. Association does not imply causation. Inferring causality requires a prospective method, a cohort study, namely recording the ACEs in much more detail as they happen and following the children into adulthood to see how their health fared. We can't imply that someone with a high ACE score *will* have adult health issues. Like other topics discussed in this book, you are not doomed by early-life trauma. One often hears stories about prominent people's early lives suggesting they had much adversity, yet they seemed to have done very well later on. Resilience and close personal relationships can buffer adversity and such afflictions can lead to positive experiences, as we see later in this chapter.

There is no prescription for a pill that will give you resilience. Nor is there any surgical procedure that can remove the effects of early-life trauma. Trauma is complex and takes years, if not a lifetime, to heal from. Felitti feels that acknowledgment of ACEs is the first step in therapy. Trauma-informed care is another treatment to consider. Trauma-informed care involves providing teachers, social workers, mental health practitioners, physicians, and others who work with traumatized clients or patients with the knowledge and tools to understand and treat someone whose cognitive, behavioral, and psychosocial skills have been impacted by a traumatic experience or series of such experiences.

Trauma treatment also requires societal or political changes. Bessel van der Kolk, who has written a US bestseller on trauma, writes [125]:

When I give presentations on trauma and trauma treatment, participants sometimes ask me to leave out the politics and confine myself to talking about neuroscience and therapy. I wish I could separate trauma from politics, but as long as we continue to live in denial and treat only trauma while ignoring its origins, we are bound to fail.

Exposure to harsh, brutal, or cruel parenting as a child has been explored as a force that makes one more prone to support authoritarian or aggressive policies such as foreign wars, punitive laws, and the death penalty [126,127]. Physical punishment in childhood may be a marker of a dysfunctional family environment, and researchers have explored whether this physical trauma and dysfunction lead to opposition to abortion and support for the use of military force. An argument can be made that harsh parenting in the United States may be in part responsible for America's many wars, the overturning of abortion rights, maintaining the death penalty, accepting a "strongman" leader, and many other traumatic policies [128]. Harsh parenting plays a role in pain, as well.

Chronic pain has become common today. Pain can be seen in many varieties, two of which are physical pain and social pain. Social pain as discussed in this book can be emotional, psychological, or psychic pain, among others. Chronic physical pain has been linked to attachment issues. A study of children with severe burns showed that their security of attachment to their mothers predicted the amount of morphine required to control their pain [129]. Future posttraumatic stress disorder (PTSD) in these children was also inversely linked with feeling safe with their mothers. Unlike mortality measures of health, which was the focus of my book *Inequality Kills Us All*, comparing countries on factors such as pain and attachment is more complicated. Attachment becomes more insecure, due to the US having no national paid maternity leave, as discussed above; this lack of attachment leads to more pain, likely of the social variety [130]. This widespread pain helps explain why the United States consumes most of the world's opioids. US drug companies were promoting opioid drugs as nonaddictive pain medicines; however, this practice has stopped while opioid drug deaths are at record levels. This situation, and the association of nonsuicidal self-injury with ACEs, is discussed further in the mental health chapter (Chapter 7).

Since ACEs, or childhood trauma, figure so prominently in adult health outcomes, what about international comparisons of ACEs, while still recognizing their shortcomings mentioned earlier? Our health Olympics, discussed further in the next chapter, looks at deaths among nations where they are usually accurately tabulated and elsewhere where they are estimated to some precision. Tabulating ACEs and trauma among nations is more complex. A review of studies provides estimates of the proportion of various populations, such as students, older adults, and less specific groups, having two or more ACEs using a 10-item questionnaire [131]. Another study of 28 nations found high numbers of ACEs and called for both upstream and downstream interventions. Adverse childhood experiences often precede not only poor health but also adverse behavioral outcomes [132]. Intergenerational transmission of trauma is common [133,134]. Studies show high levels in the US and among minority groups. We must recognize that ACEs are likely to be underreported, so the impacts may be greater.

Having more ACEs also leads to worse oral health, based on measurements such as the number of missing or decayed teeth [135]. Adverse childhood experiences and dental health are also impacted by income inequality; some additional health effects of income inequality will be explored in the next chapter.

Expect much more to be learned about the profound impact of childhood trauma on various societal outcomes. Substantial economic costs to a nation result from their inhabitants experiencing ACEs. The impact of trauma on the developing brain of a child can produce an adult with disrupted thought processes and limited impulse control. Adversity in early life is bad for population health [136].

With these studies and findings in mind, pieces of the puzzle seem to fit. But there's one more piece to consider. Trauma does not always end badly, or rather, trauma can be healed.

POSTTRAUMATIC GROWTH

Posttraumatic growth (PTG) refers to situations whereby those who have had ACEs, PTSD, or another form of trauma experience positive changes resulting from their struggles [137].

Posttraumatic growth is a process and an outcome, namely the experience of positive changes through the struggle with traumatic events. In contrast to resilience, which refers to recovering from illness or trauma, PTG is a transformative response that results in a new level of improved functioning. One's beliefs about how the world works and rumination over the trauma can lead to acceptance of the changed world and being further ahead than before the hardship.

The United States has more than its share of trauma: losing wars with disastrous numbers of casualties, mass shootings, and other forms of violence, not to overlook our poor outcomes in early life. Yet I'm not suggesting we should celebrate our poor health outcomes as creating conditions for PTG. Negative experiences can often foster the recognition of one's personal strength. They can lead to exploring new possibilities, as well as improving relationships, leading to spiritual growth [138].

Many factors can facilitate PTG. One is finding an expert companion to listen, tolerate, and be there. Such a person can take the pressure off you. There are vast cultural differences in this process and there are no predictable stages. Action, instead of or in addition to talk, may be required. Psychotherapy and other clinical interventions may also help you emerge stronger. Interaction with an animal companion is another way of intervening to foster PTG. This has been studied with US veterans by organizations using dogs and horses to improve quality of life [139].

Beyond ACEs and other forms of psychic and physical injury, it's access to resources that remains a key factor in mediating all the consequences stemming from early life.

EFFECTS OF POVERTY

How can societies have policies that support early life? Earlier we learned that, for most of human existence on Earth, poverty, as we know it today, was absent. People shared scarce resources, namely food. With the development of agriculture, hierarchies emerged, together with deprivation, with some having less than needed to survive. Over 500 years ago, "poor laws" and houses for paupers were developed in England as a way to deal with beggars. Helping the poor was a way to justify taxation to assist the aged, handicapped, and worthy poor. The "unworthy" poor, deemed to be lazy and unwilling to pull themselves up by their bootstraps, were not helped, but were put into workhouses. The moral hazard argument, which says that if you help those poor, they won't seek employment, is well discredited [140]. With the advent of the welfare state in Great Britain after World War II, however, there was a change in the way people understood poverty and disadvantage, and a challenge to the moral hazard argument. Poor laws have mostly disappeared, but the notion that some people are more worthy and entitled to having their basic needs met than others remains, which perpetuates poverty, and the toleration of poverty, and its adverse impact on health.

Cross-national studies using fetal ultrasounds and looking at poverty in France, the Netherlands, Norway, Spain, Sweden, the United Kingdom, and the United States found smaller fetuses by the second trimester among impoverished households [141]. Low-resourced parents have fetuses with decreased brain volumes, that is less gray matter, which has been associated with compromised developmental outcomes later in life [96]. Markers of stress are also more commonly seen among economically marginalized and exploited communities – otherwise termed the poor. Such parents who are stressed in their early lives may have newborns with altered brain development [142].

Impoverishing vulnerable families and households and leaving them without adequate social safety nets is a policy – and thus political – choice, but acceptance of this concept varies around the world. Census bureau data show increasing numbers living in poverty. International comparisons show the US typically has among the highest child poverty and hunger poverty of all rich nations [143]. The United States is said to be a meritocracy, namely our society is based on the premise that everyone in America can achieve great things based on their merit. Inherent in this myth is the assumption that people succeed because they've worked hard, and if they are poor then it is their own fault for not working hard enough [144].

As this chapter has shown, early life shapes adult health, and a multitude of those adverse early-life effects are directly related to having limited individual, family, and community access and entitlement to resources, which is poverty [145]. The obscene wealth gap in the United States is a strong indicator of our nation's inequality. Depending on how wealth is assessed, the richest 1% of Americans have as much or more wealth than the bottom half of people in the country, in some cases considerably more. This condition is termed excessive wealth disorder. Excessive wealth disorder results from how the rich have gamed the system to have more than anyone else. Consider immiseration – the misery of resource deprivation that is the result of intentional, avoidable policies of exploitation, greed, and meanness – as inequality's conjoined twin. More on that later, but first let's explore the influence of income and wealth inequality on population health.

CHAPTER FIVE

Economic Inequality Is Bad for Our Health

The form of law which I propose would be as follows: In a state which is desirous of being saved from the greatest of all plagues – not faction, but rather distraction – there should be among the citizens neither extreme poverty nor, again, excessive wealth, for both are productive of great evil.

Plato

Income inequality is a social cancer, and poverty, its twin, is also a carcinogen, as suggested by Dr. Samuel Broder, the director of the National Cancer Institute [146]. Like cancer, we generally first become aware of income inequality through subtle signs. Then it can spread, intensify, and erode your body, as a malignancy does. Consider your personal experiences with inequality beginning with your earliest memories. Wherever you grew up within the economic hierarchy, you no doubt discovered at some point that some people were better off, and others worse off, than your family. I learned about inequality as a young child growing up in a working-class community in Toronto, Canada, in the 1940s and 1950s. My father repaired shoes and we lived above the shoe repair store. Our neighbors similarly worked hard and there were few status differences among us. One distinction I remember was a professional wrestler who lived somewhere in the neighborhood and drove a pink Cadillac convertible, which became a marker of his status, in comparison to that of my family and other families that relied on public transportation.

In the public schools I attended, most of the students were similarly working class and I did not feel out of place. Nor were there big differences attending the University of Toronto, beginning in 1962. It wasn't until 1966, when I went to Harvard University in Cambridge, Massachusetts, that

I became acutely aware of class differences. I had expected everyone would be well-dressed, but was really surprised by how privileged people would dress down to show their status – they didn't need to impress. I later became a resident tutor in Dunster House, 1 of the 12 undergraduate dormitories. I lived among these wealthy students, one of whom later became the US vice president. Surrounded by these privileged students, I hid my humble beginnings, my social cancer, from my undergraduate charges who would later achieve such prominence.

Spending a year in Nepal, however, suddenly cast me as entitled, compared with those in the hillside peasant villages I trekked through. Caste, considered a ritual hereditary class system in Hindu society, is an inherent part of Nepal, with Brahmins, the priestly caste, occupying the highest rank. Those who worked with leather were of a very low caste, *Sarki*, which, given my father was a shoe repairman, was my caste. When I said I was a Sarki no one would believe me. "You couldn't be a Sarki!" they'd exclaim, assuming I must not understand the meaning of that caste label, given the abundance I presented, such as my camera. Yet for me, my identity as a Sarki was one I felt deep in my bones, having always known that, despite my Harvard education, I had come from the class of leather-workers. In Hindu villages, when amongst Nepali Brahmins who did not know I was a Sarki, I could not enter their homes as, being a foreigner, I would pollute them. I typically slept in an animal shed. It was like being ritually excluded when among the Boston Brahmins while a student at Harvard. I internalized this sense of status at Harvard, which was not then coeducational, when I dated a woman who went to Radcliffe. Knowing her privilege, I never told her about my working-class background.

I then went on to Stanford medical school and gained status as a doctor. My life's upward-bound trajectory has been rooted in my good fortune of getting higher education degrees from prestigious universities. I used my social cancer to advantage. To impress people in casual conversations, I might mention having degrees from Harvard, Stanford, and Johns Hopkins, and these pedigreed degrees would certainly open doors that would not have opened for me without them. But deep down, my malignancy kept me a working-class dude, even if no one else knew.

In the early 1970s, doctors were mostly White, male, and from privileged backgrounds. Though unusual for that time, some African Americans and women were admitted to Stanford. Most of our professors were White and male. And their wives were more often nurses than other doctors. Nurses marrying doctors was a form of upward mobility for women that is today much less common. In many medical schools today, however, women form the majority of medical students. Today, male doctors often marry female doctors.

Today, status differences for most people are affirmed in early life by social media and the internet, which provide the means of continuously comparing oneself to others. Status is marked by looks, dress, and numerous affectations. Besides education, incomes can be discerned. Although asking someone's income is not a polite topic of conversation in the United States, it is in South Asia. For faculty members in a state school system, every employee's income can be found on the internet. Once I looked up mine and that of others, I did not like discovering how some colleagues made much more than I did. Suddenly, the impressive income I earned felt paltry. I never repeated the inspection. Status comparisons inevitably leave us feeling subordinate. Even as we promote our successes and status on social media, we come away feeling less good than we perceive others to be. There are many ways people internalize and otherwise respond to inequalities in society, especially those of income and wealth. Some fall into depression. Others express frustration toward their partners for not earning enough. Some even plunge into significant debt, purchasing luxury cars, oversized homes, designer clothes, and indulging in extravagant vacations they can't afford, all to impress others. Ironically, this pursuit leads some to bankruptcy.

Alfred Adler, the Austrian psychoanalyst, spoke of the "inferiority complex," suggesting it is an innate part of being human today [147]. He argued that people respond to their inferiority with shyness or low self-esteem or by hiding their insecurity by trying to conquer others through many means, including violence. These efforts vary among societies. Weddings provide an example. Eschewing tradition, my first was modest by today's lavish standards portrayed in the media. My last, marrying someone who grew up on a farm, was downright cheap, as it reflected our combined values of avoiding excess.

As inequality increases within nations, those rich enough can afford the increased prices luxury brands charge. Others go to dollar stores or go into debt to enjoy a few prestige items. Egyptian tombs present an archaeological display of wealth. Throughout human history, large status differences have always resulted in almost everyone having an inferiority complex – even the rich feel inferior for not being the richest [148].

We live in an age of insecurity. For the most part, the wealthy hide their feelings of insecurity from outside scrutiny [149]. The Easterlin paradox speaks to the finding that although, within countries, wealthier people are, on average, happier than poorer ones [150], across countries and over time, increases in per capita income do not produce more happiness, as we saw in Chapter 1. Much evidence suggests that, for the rich, their wealth does not bring them more joy [151]. On occasion, well-to-do Nepali doctors from the urban capital, Kathmandu, would have to hike up into the surrounding hills. They typically found this trek very arduous and would be passed on the hillside by peasant farmers running barefoot over the rocks, laughing while carrying huge loads. These privileged people would ask me, "How can I be struggling so much when they seem so exhilarated?"

It could be argued that the increase in house sizes is a sign of this insecurity. Karl Marx said, "A house may be large or small; as long as the surrounding houses are equally small, it satisfies all social demands for a dwelling. But if a palace rises beside the little house, the little house shrinks into a hut." [152]. The house I own today was purchased from a family whose earner was a downtown department store delivery-man and is more than adequate. However, McMansions have sprouted around my hut!

IS INEQUALITY THE MOTHER OF ALL EVILS?

The ravages of inequality can be found in the *Laws* of Plato from the fourth century BCE. Plato's limit for a healthy society prescribes the wealthiest to have no more than four times that of the least wealthy. The ratio today, however, is stratospheric.

We considered the modern-day equivalent of plagues in Chapter 3, when discussing the studies linking income inequality to health outcomes as measured by mortality across countries, which were first published in 1979. A few studies followed but escaped attention until 1992, when the paper "Income distribution and life expectancy," by Richard Wilkinson, was published [153]. Wilkinson graphed the income received by the least well-off 70% of a country's families against their life expectancy for the nine rich nations. A striking correlation appeared: populations in countries with the greatest inequality face a life expectancy that is three years lower than that in the countries that are most equal. Looking at trends (health tends to improve over time), he also demonstrated that increases in relative poverty levels over time are associated with smaller life expectancy improvements.

The study led to two 1996 investigations demonstrating the inequality–mortality relationship across US states [154,155]. A 1998 study considered income distributions and mortality rates in US cities [156]. Across cities, whether richer or poorer, less inequality was related to lower mortality rates. The highest mortality rates were seen in the cities with large income gaps, suggesting that relative inequality matters more for mortality than being richer or poorer.

Compare mortality rates and income inequality in Canada's 10 provinces with those in the 50 US states [157]. The 10 Canadian provinces' mortality and inequality data points are grouped with only four of the best-performing US states. The tilt of the line linking the Canadian provinces was less steep than that for the US states (Figure 5.1). Income inequality matters less in Canada than in the United States. Why? In the US, people live in a cafeteria society. If you want something, you have to pay for it. Very little is provided to Americans, as exemplified by there not being a national law for paid maternity leave. Canada provides much more for its inhabitants that they don't have to pay for out of pocket. Examples include healthcare, low-cost higher education, housing support, and many other basic needs that Americans have to finance out of their incomes. Many of these costs represent social expenditures, which are quite limited in the US. Another study that looked at so-called labor market income in Canada compared with the United States found that your paycheck mattered more for your health in the US than in Canada for the same reasons [158].

Canada has a very large proportion of immigrants among its residents, some 50% more than in the US. The inequality–health relationship in Canada is not there for immigrants, but it exists for those born in Canada [159]. That study followed two million Canadians over the last decade of the past century. The authors recorded their mortality rates and incomes and found no impact of income inequality on the mortality of immigrants, unlike for those native-born. Reasons may include the strong

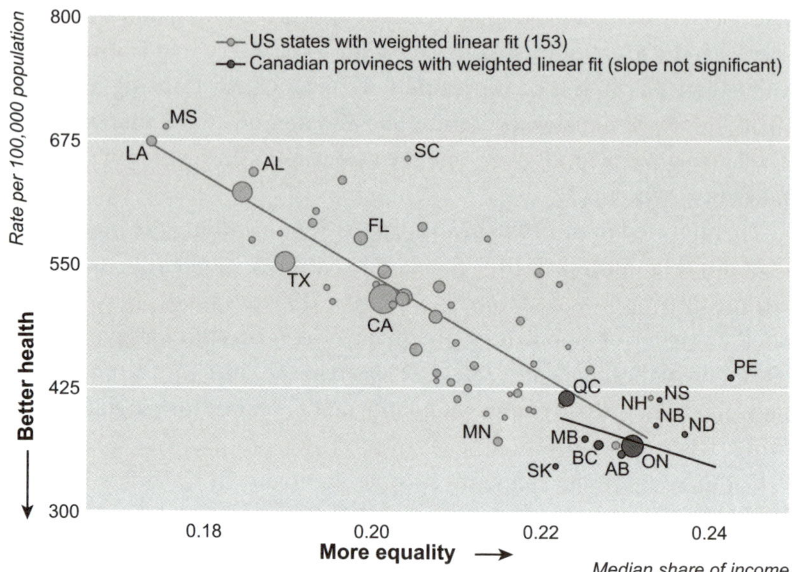

5.1 Mortality among working-age men, USA and Canada [157]

support immigrants give to others from abroad [160]. One can go on and on summarizing many studies pointing out that inequality is bad for our health.

There are some situations where the relationship between income inequality and health is weak or not found. Examples such as presented above for Canada, where there is a stronger social safety net and fewer effects from inequality, are also found in populations called welfare states. The size of the community matters too. We tend to live among our peers. So, in a small population, the income gap may not be very big. What determines health outcomes in small areas is the average income there. Richer communities have better health than poorer ones. This speaks to the concept of deprivation relative to the rest of society. More economically deprived areas have worse health. There appears to be an inequality threshold that has to be breached before the relationship is seen in statistical studies.

The Spirit Level: Why More Equal Societies Almost Always Do Better, by Richard G. Wilkinson and Kate Pickett, appeared in 2009 [161]. The title, chosen by the publisher in the United Kingdom, relates to the spirit level, which we call a carpenter's level here. The less forceful subtitle of the US edition was *Why Greater Equality Makes Societies Stronger*. A bestseller and translated into many languages, Wilkinson and Pickett's book has made an important impact.

Their genius is how they produced a key graph, Figure 5.2. Country income inequality measures are on the horizontal axis and range from low to high, without numbers to confuse the concept. On the vertical axis is an index of multiple health and social problems, which are listed to the left of the graph. Twenty-one rich countries are scattered in the graph lying close to a line relating the health and social problems index to income inequality. The problems listed are life expectancy, math and literacy scores, infant mortality, homicides, imprisonment, teenage births, trust, obesity, mental illness, and social mobility. Details with the actual numbers are in the book's appendix.

Japan, on the lower left, has the best outcomes and lowest income inequality while the United States stands at the opposite end with the

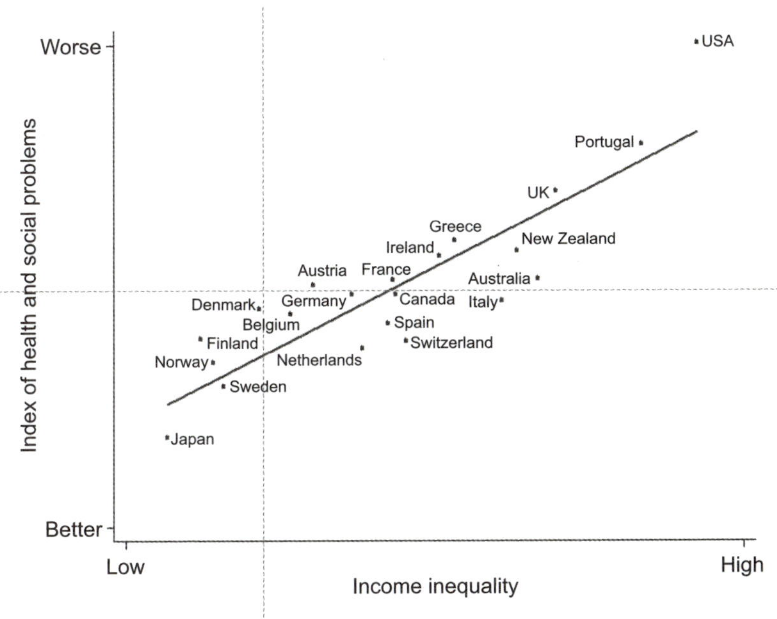

5.2 Health and social problems related to income inequality [161]

highest income inequality and worst outcomes. Besides mostly supportive reviews, the book's publication led to some disparate rejoinders, criticisms, and screeds not based on scientific principles. In an updated edition the authors directly addressed those and many other critiques in a postscript titled, *Research Meets Politics.*

What about wealth? Wealth data are elusive, so there are fewer studies. Wealth inequality is far greater than income inequality [162]. The existing rich-country studies do support wealth inequality impacting health. The wealth of American adults at midlife is associated with longer lives. Intergenerational transfer of wealth may have a more profound effect on health than wealth accumulated in one's lifetime [163].

A European study looked at self-rated health and life satisfaction in 28 countries [164]. In a culturally similar population, self-assessed health mirrors mortality measures. More income inequality leads to poorer health and lower life satisfaction. The research pointed out that inequality has well-being costs for wealthy people as well as for impoverished people. Neighborhood problems (noise, congestion, air pollution, litter) in more unequal countries increase with increasing income, in contrast to more equal countries where problems decrease with increasing income (demonstrating effect modification or interaction for biostatisticians). The researchers argue that, in a more unequal society, increasing private income cannot mitigate the social and environmental limitations of a sociopolitically unequal society.

Hundreds of analyses support the "greater inequality, worse health" relationship. A 15-year update of the data in *The Spirit Level* presents many more outcomes [165,166]. The relationships appear stronger, together with income inequality increasing during that interval. Despite the 2009 far-reaching report, inequality has not contracted, but risen considerably.

One of the world's premiere journals to publish science-related research is *Science.* The May 23, 2014, issue had a special section "The Science of Inequality" featuring news and research that highlights many of the ideas presented in this book.

Consider studies that look at inequality and violence.

VIOLENCE AND INEQUALITY

Homicides have been linked to income inequality through many studies [167]. The recent increases in US firearm violence are related to the rich–poor gap [168]. Police killings are also associated with income inequality [169]. Increasing income inequality decreases people's trust in one another, as seen across nations and within US states. Trust in institutions follows similar patterns. As inequality has risen spectacularly in the US, Americans' trust in their government is at an all-time low. With the decline in interpersonal and organizational trust, some people take matters into their own hands through violent means such as using guns.

One finds a considerable gender gap in gun violence, with men offending much more than women. Gender norm stereotypes are changing more quickly for women than for men. Women are achieving more status and respect today, which makes some men feel threatened. Strained masculinity can emerge with differing outcomes, including acts of violence [170]. One perspective on being a man today requires displays of violence (sometimes learned through internet gaming [171]), power, and control over others to confirm one's maleness. Mass shootings have become common and increasingly deadlier in the United States, and are almost always perpetrated by males.

A mass shooting is more likely to take place in US counties with both high income inequality and high incomes [172]. Such an explanation for what has become so customary in America will not be found in the mainstream media, where there is much self-censorship. While economic inequality is often mentioned in news reports, its link to health outcomes is not.

The United States is not the only country where mass shootings occur. However, a large proportion of them occur in the US. Firearm availability is a major factor, with far more guns than people in the US. There are more assault rifles in the hands of civilians than in the military. No other nation has a higher gun ownership rate. These statistics reflect America's national gun culture, said to be enshrined in the Second Amendment to the US Constitution. States with more restrictive gun laws have fewer mass shooting deaths, so restricting access to guns, particularly high-powered ones such as the AR-15, which can cause mass casualties in seconds, is likely to reduce gun violence.

Violence is just one factor contributing to our early deaths that is associated with income inequality. But we die earlier than people in other nations owing to a multitude of factors. Let's take a closer look at the mortality data. What can international comparisons tell us?

HEALTH OLYMPICS

When we rank countries by life expectancy using 2022 data from the 2024 United Nations (UN) Human Development Report, we find the United States ranks behind 43 other nations in how long we live [173]. Those longer-lifespan nations include not only all the other rich nations, but also Chile, China, Czechia (the Czech Republic), Slovenia, and Thailand, which you may not consider paragons of health. The UN list excludes countries not recognized by that agency such as Taiwan, Monaco, and others where people enjoy longer lives than Americans. But our relatively short lifespan hasn't always been the case. As noted in Chapter 1, the US ranked among the top 5 or 10 nations back in the early 1950s. Its life expectancy now is about where it was in 1996, when it ranked in the 20s. Over the last few years, American life expectancy has declined absolutely, and would have done so even if COVID-19 had not increased the mortality rate. Increasing inequality shares much of the blame. Figure 5.3 shows the rankings of the top 45 nations for 2022.

Life expectancy years on the vertical axis represent the average number of years people in a country would live if the mortality rates didn't change from what they were in 2022. Consider the almost seven-year difference in life expectancy between the US and Japan, the country with the longest-lived population. For 2022, the three leading causes of death in the US were heart disease, cancer, and unintentional injuries, in that order. If the top three causes of death were eliminated and the other disease mortality rates remained unchanged, we would gain nearly seven years of life expectancy and be quite close to Japan's length of life. The health gap is huge and much more significant than spending a few more years vegetating in a nursing home.

One way to consider US health, compared with that in other countries, asks how long it will take for American health to improve to the current level of the others, assuming health does improve. Using life expectancy as the measure and looking at recent rates of improvement before health

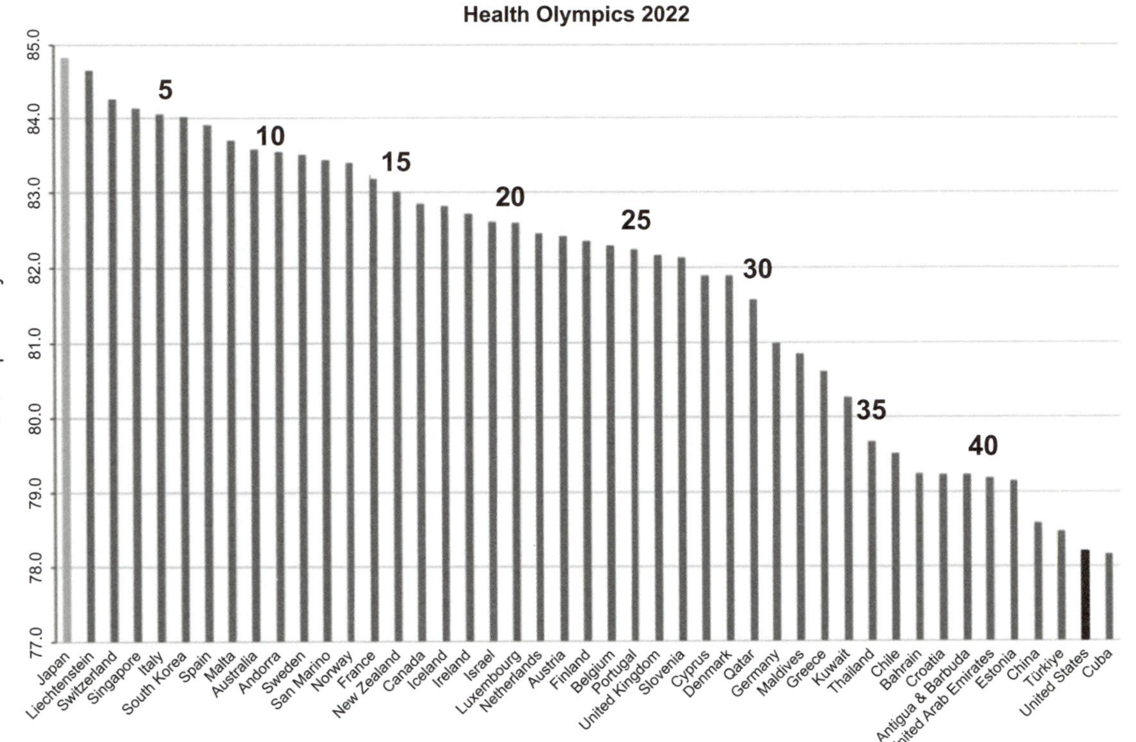

5.3 Ranking of top 45 countries by life expectancy (produced by author using data from [173])

started to decline, the time ranges from three to four decades. Compared with the 1950s, the best health outcomes have receded so much that it will take a long time to get to where the top health performers are today! If Americans really understood this, would they accept it?

Suppose we knew that in some 20 or more other countries people had smartphones, but they would not be available in the US for another 30 years. Would you tolerate that? No! You would be outraged and do something to get those devices. Our health gap is the same, only Americans don't know it. Therein lies the challenge: to make people in the United States aware they are dead first.

If health were an Olympic event, as my concept of the Health Olympics suggests, the United States would not even be there for the final race. We would have been disqualified in the trials. Knowing this, we would do something about it. In 1957 Russia launched Sputnik, the first satellite, into space, an achievement that caught America totally unprepared. That shame initiated the space race, with the US making it a goal to land a human on the Moon by the end of the 1960s. This step was an unqualified success.

The Olympic ranking in Figure 5.3 presents the United States in the best possible light. Our Central Intelligence Agency (CIA) has a world rankings website that includes a ranking for life expectancy. So does the World Bank, the World Health Organization, and others. Each of them situates the US lower than the UN report does because they recognize other nations.

INCOME INEQUALITY AND DISEASES

Income inequality and disease outcomes are another causal link in the harms faced by the unfairness caused by hierarchy. One major disease outcome found in wealthier countries, heart failure, is increasing around the world, consistent with the transition from diseases of young bowels to diseases of old arteries. With heart failure (congestive heart failure), the heart can't pump blood adequately to meet the body's needs. Researchers from Canada, Denmark, France, Norway, Sweden, the UK, and the US looked at heart failure among people in 54 countries and related it to income inequality [174]. Higher income inequality in a nation was associated with worse outcomes for heart failure, namely requiring hospital admission or death. More adverse health conditions, such as obesity, coronary heart disease, and high blood pressure, are found in developed and developing countries that have greater income inequality. Greater income inequality in US states predicted higher risks of dying from coronary heart disease and suicide. Such findings, sometimes referred to as a fundamental cause approach, call for a "health in all policies" strategy to achieve population health. We conclude that health outcomes are related to societal, structural, and psychosocial issues related to inequality.

Oral health also remains a significant problem around the world. It stands to reason that people lacking income and resources have bad dental health, including decayed, missing, or filled teeth, periodontal or gum disease, and less use of available dental care. However, where there is more income inequality, oral health outcomes are worse, both at the country level and within nations [175]. Stress, poor diet, and lack of access to dental care (all arguably symptomatic of a society with high income inequality) play major roles in poor oral health.

STRESS IS THE TWENTY-FIRST-CENTURY TOBACCO

Americans don't smoke cigarettes much anymore and now have one of the lowest rates of smoking of any nation. However, replacing the bad effect of smoking is chronic stress, the major element in the psychosocial pathway for how inequality leads to worse health. Inequality has corrosive effects on society, leading to the loss of social capital. Whether as individuals or in communities, social capital leads to connections with others that we can call on for help or cooperation [68]. Myriad mechanisms relating to social status may be at work. However, through status competition we lose social capital or cohesion, and individualism takes its place. This loss leads to a focus on individual identity politics. Society suffers. When there is less social cohesion, induced by greater income inequality, it leads to more chronic stress. The United States is one of the most stressed countries in the world, despite all the wealth and technology that should make life easier. There are environmental impacts of inequality that are eroding our health, too.

ENVIRONMENTAL IMPACTS OF INEQUALITY

The state of the global environment and the climate catastrophe are also related to inequality. Markers of planetary health, such as CO_2 and other greenhouse gases, municipal waste, and recycling, are worse in more unequal nations. Business leaders in more equal countries are more likely to comply with international environmental agreements. People in more equal countries are more likely to engage in behaviors that have environmental benefits, such as recycling waste materials.

A US study looked at political power distribution, the environment, and public health in the 50 states [176]. The researchers used various measures to represent the factors considered. Measures related to pollution, toxic chemicals, waste production, and workplace conditions, among many other things. Outcomes studied included infant mortality and premature death. They found that income inequality, impoverishment, and being racialized as a person of color led to worse health outcomes. Inequality is bad not only for our health, but also for the environment. Air pollution affects us all, but people with lower incomes and people of color usually bear the heaviest burden of negative changes in the environment due to environmental racism and race- and class-stratified zoning laws, living conditions and neighborhoods, and enforcement of environmental protections.

Consider the harmful health effects of air pollution around the globe. Particulate matter in the atmosphere, fine inhalable chemicals of less than 2.5 microns in diameter (30 times smaller than a strand of human hair), causes a host of health problems (including heart attacks, strokes, congestive heart failure, asthma, and other respiratory disorders) when inhaled. The adverse health impacts of breathing equal amounts of these fine particles are more detrimental to people living in states with higher income gaps [177]. Their worse outcomes result from many factors inherent in environmental injustice that influences their pathology. Income inequality is bad for all of us, but does not affect us all to the same extent.

INEQUALITY AND BUFFERS

US federalism devolves any powers not directly within the purview of the federal government (the executive branch, Congress, and the Supreme

Court) to the state. The US states have considerable latitude in their assorted policies that impact human welfare and the environment. State policies and policy domains range from liberal to conservative, with states characterized as liberal being more likely to have favorable environmental policies, as well as having longer life expectancies.

What role does income inequality play among the US states and their health outcomes? One study showed that states with greater income inequality have more conservative state policies and lower life expectancy [178]. In that study, California and New York have liberal state policies and quite high income inequality. Nonetheless, both states have higher life expectancy. The study presented three views on why income inequality undermines health. The first, the psychosocial perspective, relates inferiority, voiced by Adler and others, to chronic stress and the lack of power. The second perspective, social capital, focuses on lack of interpersonal trust and decreasing political collective efforts. The third, neomaterialist, considers how power and wealth are captured by elites who act in their own self-interest. The three are not mutually exclusive and reinforce each other. Similarly, the liberal–conservative policy domains form a continuum to mediate or moderate the effect of income inequality. There was less effect of income inequality at the state level where there were more liberal political policies in place. The researchers' conclusions are to take both the following actions at the state level: decrease income inequality and enact more liberal state policies. Investing in different health promotion and welfare programs can only buffer the effects of high income inequality.

OTHER HARMS OF INEQUALITY

Inequality is about political power over resources and the unjust distribution of both power and resources. There can be direct power, such as wielded by the US president, who (using executive orders whose legality can be questioned) is at liberty to invade other nations and kill millions of people, such as we've seen in Afghanistan, Iraq, and Vietnam. Another form of power is agenda setting, the ability to keep discussion on or off the table, influenced by the many types of media. Most Americans would like to see inequality decrease or to have a single-payer healthcare system. Yet these achievable goals are not on the order of business. Another is framing power, the capacity to make the outlandish seem reasonable and the unappealing seem desirable. Tax cuts for the rich are an example. They are presented as good for everyone. I'm reminded of a cartoon by David Sipress in which a banker and a worker are in a bar. The worker says to the banker, "As a potential lottery winner, I totally support tax cuts for the wealthy."

Power has been called the ultimate aphrodisiac. Power is most effective when least observable. Those with great power prefer to see their power as conferred by the market or ordained by God. And those of us with less or no power prefer to not see ourselves as subject to forces beyond our control.

Tony Benn, who was a Member of Parliament in Britain for 47 years, had five questions to ask a powerful person [179]. "What power have you got? Where did you get it from? In whose interests do you exercise it? To whom are you accountable? And how can we get rid of you?" He maintained that if you cannot get rid of the people who govern you, you do not live in a democratic system.

Big corporations have the most power in the US, and increasingly around the world. Corporate CEO pay has skyrocketed – now close to 1,000 times that of the least paid (recall Plato recommended a maximum gap of four to one) – and there is no serious intent to lower it. Instead, there is discussion of increasing the minimum wage. This won't do much, as the maximum wage will continue to rise. We cannot get rid of corporations, and thus we should question whether we have a true democracy. For example, we do not have proportional representation, which is typically considered to be required for a democracy. Each state gets two senators. Wyoming, with fewer than a million people, has the same number representing them (two) as do the over 40 million people living in California. And the US electoral college system, left over from our human enslavement history to keep the Southern States in the Union, allows the president to take office without a majority of the vote. Meanwhile, gerrymandering congressional districts has led to widely skewed representation favoring those in power, not those who vote.

Consider inequality as a highly toxic odorless, colorless, invisible gas of which we are almost entirely unaware, which kills us through the usual diseases or trauma. Inequality is not a natural outcome of disproportionate merit, as we've been led to believe. It is a policy choice, just like our perpetuation and tolerance of so many fellow humans living in poverty. Corporations responsible for this inequality are getting away with murder. This structural violence is much more harmful than the many forms of individual violence mentioned earlier in this chapter. Corporate crime pays very well. One example is Purdue Pharma, the company that marketed opioids as not addictive and made billions of dollars [180]. Millions were killed but no one from the company nor the owners, the Sackler family, went to jail. Instead, they paid fines which paled in comparison to the profits they killed for.

DEATHS OF DESPAIR

Deaths of despair refers to the original finding that American White men aged 45 to 54 have seen their mortality increase from drugs, alcohol, and suicide. With the exodus of manufacturing jobs, which began in the 1970s when the automobile and steel factories closed and moved to developing countries where wages were lower and labor and environmental laws more lax, the White working class experienced rapid economic immiseration. Having once been able to find well-paying jobs with good health-care insurance and lifetime job security – work that could support a family on a single wage – these high-school-educated White workers found themselves employable only in the lowest-paying jobs, with minimal to no benefits or job security.

The first such study found rises in mortality among US White people. This was not seen among Latinx nor among those from Australia, Canada, France, Germany, Sweden, or the United Kingdom. Subsequent research demonstrated that rising deaths were concentrated among less educated men and women across the board, including African Americans. For those without a college degree, deaths of despair occurred at rates three times higher than those with a BA [181]. At the US county level, more income inequality together with lack of social mobility led to higher rates of deaths of despair. Consider American mass shootings as murders of despair. These conditions of anguish are now seen elsewhere. A Canadian study found income inequality was related to deaths of despair (suicide, drug overdose, and alcoholic liver disease) and all-cause deaths among youths aged 20 years and younger [182].

For everyone in the US between the ages of 15 and 60, mortality is now considerably higher than in peer nations: Australia, Austria, Belgium, Canada, Denmark, Finland, France, Germany, Italy, Japan, Norway, Portugal, Spain, Sweden, Switzerland, and the UK [183]. The death ratio peaks at age 25 to be 2.5 times higher in the US than in these other countries. The chance of dying for a 25-year-old in the United States is more than 2.5 times higher than the average in the abovementioned countries [184]. The primary causes of these deaths are drugs and alcohol, deaths of self-medication. Besides deaths of despair, other causes of early death are cardiac and metabolic disorders (such as diabetes) and gun violence [185]. Unlike deaths from COVID-19, there are no signs these causes will let up.

Working-class US White men and women had once expected to achieve the American Dream, namely become richer than their parents through hard work. But this myth of meritocracy is just that – a myth. In pursuit of this unattainable myth, many people self-medicate through harmful behaviors, consuming drugs and alcohol, as well as sugar and highly processed foods, to assuage their perceived failure. Rather than remain active, as adults in other countries are more likely to do, television, video games, and social media addictions are common. People consume and engage in these addictive substances and behaviors to get dopamine, a neurotransmitter, released in their brains to feel better (more on dopamine in Chapter 7), but these compulsive activities harm them in the end. They need more and more of the addictive substances to get the dopamine reward. Some eventually take their lives through suicide. However, rather than posit deaths of despair as resulting from self-destructive behaviors, it may be more important to focus on structural factors, such as detachment from the blue-collar labor force, with consequent low social integration. This perspective puts the problem directly into the political realm.

Is inequality the real culprit here, or might inequality be good for us?

WHAT GOOD IS INEQUALITY?

Given all this inequality, could it be good for something? Here I present points of view that I do not hold. To me inequality has no merit in society. One argument voiced for a bigger gap between richer and poorer is that it provides incentives for those with less to work harder to achieve more and thereby benefit society. Once again, we're confronted with the meritocracy myth. Consider a cartoon in which a CEO is talking to a janitor with the caption, "I just work a billion times harder than you." Do those who take risks and innovate require substantial rewards to do so? We are led to believe that's the case, yet creativity is not driven by greed.

Another argument in support of inequality is that those who earn much more will invest their earnings in ways that will create more jobs and opportunities for those with less, the so-called trickle-down effect. Consider highly profitable companies such as Apple. It uses its vast profits to buy back its stock to increase shareholder value, rather than investing in innovation and more jobs. When supply of a stock falls, that is there are fewer shares of the stock available due to buyback, prices of the stock go up. Such a practice was illegal before 1982, but a law was passed then allowing buybacks without government scrutiny. The practice has now become commonplace, especially after the Trump-era tax cuts of 2017 that led to corporations saving vast amounts on taxes which they used to repurchase their own stock, while social expenditures were drastically cut. The rising tide has lifted the yachts but swamped the rowboats.

We've been conditioned to believe that inequality is supposed to be good for economic growth. Yet even the International Monetary Fund, among many others, has spoken out against that concept [186]. The opposite is true, with more economic growth where there is more equality. Economic growth in the United States has slowed while inequality has soared.

Consider economic inequality as a market failure. Firms tend toward monopolies that concentrate power and can set higher prices to gain more profits. This also leads to workers being paid less, which increases inequality. This vicious cycle is difficult to break.

Given all these negative aspects of greater inequality, not to mention the key messages about worse health and so many adverse societal factors (such as the social problems index above), why does it exist? The rich and powerful have always wanted only one thing: more! They have crafted policies to get more. Yet ultimately, this does not benefit them, as they are neither that healthy nor happy, and nor are the rest of us.

DOES INEQUALITY *CAUSE* WORSE HEALTH?

I have implied that income and wealth inequality cause worse health. But many assert that correlation is not causation. How do you decide that something causes something else? That topic is not discussed much in our educational system.

In Chapter 3 we looked at how inequality can cause worse health by making three points. To review, one finds better health outcomes among those with higher incomes. But there are diminishing returns to health improvements for those with a great deal of income when they get a tranche more. Taking income from the rich and giving it to those who are poorer improves almost everyone's health. In other words, those making a million dollars a year are unlikely to see worse health by making only $900,000.

The second issue is that a big income or wealth gap creates more stress for almost everyone. Psychosocial stress is increasing throughout the world during our current era of massive transfers of wealth to the top 1%. We suffer from an enormous amount of pain from being so stressed by the rising costs of our most basic needs – food, shelter, and healthcare.

Third, those with too much ensure they control the system so they can have even more. The 2010 Citizens United decision by the US Supreme Court allowed unlimited contributions to political campaigns. Consequently, corporations – which the Supreme Court has ruled have the same rights as people – and the wealthiest citizens – those who control business and manufacturing – can bankroll politicians. The rich game the system to their advantage. Consider the current issue of raising the debt ceiling for the US federal government. If taxes on the rich were raised, there would be no problem with debt. In the 1950s there was no need to take on federal debt, as the highest marginal tax rate was 91%. That meant that if someone making a million dollars made another dollar, he got to keep only nine cents of that dollar. That tax system was fair because millionaires could stay rich, but only so rich, before they were expected to contribute more to the society that had made them rich. Today the *lowest* combined rate of federal, state, and local taxes is paid by the richest 400 families in America [187]. This is quite a contrast to the 1960s, when the richest paid the highest rate of tax. The diametric switch resulted from the assault on taxation, which will be described in Chapter 8.

Those explanations are valid, but may not be sufficient for epidemiologists. Epidemiology is the study of diseases and factors affecting health, especially their distribution, namely who gets them and why. In the mid nineteenth century, John Snow, a British physician, began mapping cholera deaths in London. Cholera was an illness where people had profound diarrhea, leading to severe dehydration and death. Snow found that cholera cases clustered around a water pump on Broad Street. He concluded there was something about the water that caused cholera. He knew nothing about the bacterium, *Vibrio cholerae*, in the water that caused the infection. Nevertheless, he persuaded the city's leaders to remove the pump handle so no one could get water there. Deaths declined. This experiment demonstrated that you don't need to know everything about a disease or health condition to act and do the right thing. Still, even after the decline in deaths, epidemiologists were loath to infer causality.

In the 1950s, epidemiologist Austin Bradford Hill laid out criteria for deciding whether something causes something else. You need to have some evidence that demonstrates a relationship between one thing and another. An obvious example is when someone has a loaded firearm, points it at another person's heart, pulls the trigger, a hole appears, blood pours out, and the victim dies. There is a smoking gun! With income inequality, researchers discovered that, in populations with a big gap in earnings, there is worse health than in others with a small earnings gap. Notice that while there is hard evidence here, there is no smoking gun!

One of Hill's criteria is that there needs to be a dose–response situation, namely, more inequality leads to worse outcomes, or less inequality leads to better outcomes. It helps to have evidence for different groups, done by different researchers over different time periods. Consider deaths from mass shootings in different places across the United States over the last few years. No question about the smoke here. Where gun laws are more restrictive, there is less gun violence. Where gun laws are more lax, there is more gun violence. When gun laws are loosened, as we've seen in Texas, where now anyone can carry any type of firearm in public, without a permit and with no background check (with some restrictions), mass shootings have risen. Yet many people continue to claim there is no evidence that lax gun laws cause more gun violence. We might say that they've blinded themselves to the evidence, because they don't want to accept its implications – that if we had fewer guns, we'd have fewer deaths. However, it would be more accurate to say they have had the wool pulled over their eyes by a gun lobby bent on making profits by selling more and more guns by any means necessary, including stopping research at the federal level [188].

Another requirement asks what came first, the chicken or the egg? Did the person with a gun aimed at them die of a heart attack before the trigger was pulled? Or was it the other way around, namely, the trigger was pulled and the victim died of the injury? Or, for the subject of our chapter, do people get sick and then make less money than the nonsick? Or do those who make more money get less sick? A recent study of almost two million people in Ontario, Canada, looked at the neighborhood incomes of people with diabetes [189]. Of the people studied, those who lived in lower-income communities were more likely to die. No matter what killed the people with diabetes there, the study found that those living in places where people had lower incomes (i.e. there was more neighborhood disenfranchisement) were more likely to die. Another study looked at US breast cancer survival and found the same result.

Next, one had to consider whether there is a better explanation. Look again at our smoking gun example. Some could conclude that the shooter lived, because he believed in God and the victim didn't. So, the devil placed the hole in the heart, and the shooter used a starter pistol with no bullet. While these explanations might seem absurd, they aren't any more ridiculous than some make for dismissing the relationship between inequality and health. For the "more inequality, worse health" situation, are there better explanations? For example, is there more sophisticated medical care where there is less inequality, or belief in a supernatural power that produces better health? Skeptics will always find some other interpretation. This book argues for a better explanation.

The above criteria for making the claim that income inequality causes worse health outcomes was addressed in an important study mentioned in Chapter 3 [59]. That study has been cited thousands of times to mostly affirm other observations. More recent academic reviews continue to explore causality.

Other criteria for deciding something is causal is whether it is consistent with whatever else we know. Can it be tested experimentally? There can be natural experiments besides those under controlled conditions. For early-life issues, many such experiments have been documented in the previous chapter. A natural experiment is currently taking place in the United States where income and wealth inequality are both soaring, and our health is declining absolutely.

The fall of the Soviet Union was prophesied by a French demographer, Emmanuel Todd, in his 1976 book *La chute finale: Essai sur la décomposition de la sphère soviétique*; he predicted the collapse because infant mortality rates were rising among countries there [190]. After the 1991 breakup of the Soviet Union, mortality rates drastically increased in Russia, almost like the US deaths of despair described above. What happened is that the Kremlin sold the state assets to oligarchs at fire-sale prices. Inequality quickly intensified, and deaths also skyrocketed. Over 30 years later, Russia's health is about what it was in 1991.

US infant mortality has risen over the last few years, life expectancy is declining, and inequality is soaring. Will Americans face the same situation as post-Soviet Russia, although at a slower pace as our inequality has not skyrocketed quickly?

Another natural experiment with a different outcome happened in Japan when the United States occupied the country. In 1945, Japan's life expectancy was estimated to be about 24 years. The head of the allied forces occupying Japan was General Douglas MacArthur. MacArthur legislated a maximum wage for the country, broke apart the vast concentrations of wealth in the corporate conglomerates (the *zaibatsu*), and redistributed the land of this rice-farming economy from the few landowners (*jinushi*) to the peasants (*kosakumin*). There followed the most rapid decline in deaths ever seen on the planet [191]. MacArthur wrote the constitution for Japan by the equivalent of cutting and pasting in the policies of other countries. Article 9 forbade Japan to have a military; they had to resolve disputes peacefully. Today, however, the US wants Japan to develop a strong military to keep China at bay. But the Japanese like not having an army and constitutions are difficult to change. Article 23 makes the government responsible for the health of the nation. This "medicine" was so successful that, by 1978, Japan was the longest-lived nation, a standing it maintains today.

We can see that abruptly increasing income and wealth inequality is bad for health and quickly decreasing it leads to good health. Economic inequality represents a policy decision, not a natural phenomenon.

Finally, consider the relationship between health and cigarette smoking. The then US Surgeon General laid out the criteria for inferring that smoking causes worse health in his 1964 report [192]. Although it had become clear 40 years before that smoking cigarettes was bad for your health, even doctors advised smoking cigarettes to calm your nerves. They pitched certain brands as being less irritating.

Chapter 3 of the Surgeon General's report is titled, "Criteria for Judgment" and lays out five criteria: (1) the consistency of the association, (2) the strength of the association, (3) the specificity of the association, (4) the temporal relationship of the association, and (5) the coherence of the association. Coherence asks if biology explains how smoking is bad for you. Yes, there are biological mechanisms to explain what happens, not just with smoking cigarettes but with income inequality and with early life. Understanding some biology helps us to recognize the critical importance of economic inequality and early-life issues in producing health. Thus, in the next chapter, we turn to biology.

CHAPTER SIX

How Biology Matters

They [elements of biology] are the agent of social causes, of social formations that determine the nature of our productive and consumption lives, and in the end, it is only through changes in those social forces that we can get to the root problem of health.

RC Lewontin

INTRODUCTION

The key point of this book is that the political decisions of how much economic inequality is structured into or inflicted by a society and how that society supports early life are the major factors responsible for the health status of the people in that society. Ancient wisdom through various traditions validates such key concepts of producing health. In today's modern scientific era, understanding biology helps comprehend causality using established criteria from epidemiology described in the previous chapter.

The John Snow cholera example (from Chapter 5) demonstrates that one doesn't need to know all the details to act and reduce deaths and suffering. However, to convince many people today, we need to know the biology of what harms and what helps our health.

What does biology, the study of life, mean to you? Perhaps around grade 4 you were first told about cells, the basic building blocks of life organisms. Cells have an outside wall, and inside is stuff called cytoplasm, and somewhere there is a nucleus. By grade 9 you were likely exposed to cell biology in greater detail. Inside the nucleus were the genes made up of DNA residing in chromosomes. This knowledge arose from various experiments and studies.

This chapter explores the biology behind inequality as well as that of early life on adult health. Inequality increases stress levels, as does neglect in early life. Here we explore stress biology.

STRESS RESPONSE

So far, we've used the word stress often. Humans have a stress response to get us out of trouble. The modern term portrays a fight-or-flight response. While living in remote Nepal in the mid 1970s, Pema, my coworker, and I were high up on the side of a mountain enjoying a day off. Yaks had been brought by Tibetans to Dhorpatan when they settled there in the early 1960s. Most yaks were decimated by liver parasites and one survived to be let feral. We came across this magnificent yak that day. I wanted to get a close-up picture. I approached the beast holding my camera to my eye to frame the ideal shot. As I inched closer and closer, suddenly I saw the animal charging at me with his hair flying. My heart raced, I breathed furiously, turned, and ran away as fast as my muscles could propel me. Pema, on the other hand, stood his ground, faced the yak, raised his arm, and shouted loudly. The yak stopped, assessed the situation, turned around, and left. Meanwhile my heart pounded and sweat poured off me as I had survived this yak attack. I'm glad Pema knew how to deal with a charging yak. Two people responded differently to a stressor. One fled and the other was willing to fight. What happens during such a stressful event?

Activation of the stress response results from the brain sensing challenges to survival. The brain initiates a cascade of responses to prime the body to react. It activates the sympathetic nervous system, a part of the autonomic (involuntary) nervous system, almost instantaneously followed by secretion of the hormone adrenaline (epinephrine) to get the heart beating faster to send more oxygenated blood to the muscles that will save your life. Your breathing increases to provide the needed oxygen. Pupils in the eyes dilate, and other responses occur without thinking. Another hormone, cortisol, is released to stop unnecessary activities such as digestion, ovulation, or tissue repair that won't save your life at that moment.

STRESS AND UNMET BASIC SOCIOECONOMIC NEEDS. Adults lower down in the socioeconomic hierarchy, as assessed by income and education, have higher stress hormone levels when challenged with a serious threat [193]. With repeated stresses, the bodies of such people may not have the capacity to produce the full stress response described above. And once stressed, chronically underresourced bodies take longer to recover from the stressor. There are also effects on cognition. Those who have lived with much chronic stress or trauma are more likely to have adverse impacts on their ability to process information [194].

OXYTOCIN, STRESS, AND SOCIAL CAPITAL. There are also gendered differences in the stress response. Historically, human research was done by men on other men. Findings were assumed to apply to women. But health and disease issues have different gendered manifestations. Oxytocin, a neuropeptide or chemical messenger, is secreted by the pituitary gland in both men and women and has effects throughout the body, including the brain, where it is central to experiencing love and safety [195]. In women it triggers labor at the end of pregnancy, as well as the release of breast milk. It is also a signaling molecule in both men and women, responding to social interactions and stressors. During stress, oxytocin may affect women differently than it affects men. If a man, a woman, and her child face a stressful event together, the man may "fight or flee" while the woman may "tend and befriend," namely protect the child [196]. During a stressful situation, offspring must be safeguarded, something more likely done by women, especially when combined with gender role socialization, which would reinforce these gendered responses to stress.

Human evolution led to sociality and dependence on others partly through hormone production. Oxytocin has many complex beneficial behavioral and health functions and could be considered "nature's medicine" [197]. Positive early-life experiences lead to increasing oxytocin-sensing regions in the brain, which are believed to enhance altruism. In other words, there are ways in which a secure early life can contribute to a greater capacity for the expression of positive adult social behaviors.

For this reason, oxytocin is thus called a prosocial hormone. More oxytocin creates more empathy. Some call it the love hormone as it fosters attachment. Neuroeconomists, studying trust in economic transactions, have called oxytocin the "moral molecule." There are higher levels of trust in more equal societies [198].

Dogs secrete oxytocin when the owner (not a stranger) looks into their eyes, and the owner releases it too [199]. The longer the mutual gaze, the higher the rise in oxytocin levels. Pets may foster social capital (discussed in Chapter 5), and may have a health benefit for their owners.

A chemically similar hormone, vasopressin, regulates water retention and compresses arteries. It helps facilitate defense and mobilization stress responses in the body. Some research suggests that, in men, vasopressin may affect paternal behavior [65].

Both oxytocin and vasopressin may stimulate or inhibit the actions of the other, allowing many variations in stress responses. Humans function best in a secure *social* environment. Without social capital, oxytocin levels in humans may decline, leaving us with less protection from stress.

CORTISOL. Cortisol, a hormone essential for many of life's vital processes, increases as part of the body's stress response to shut down unnecessary bodily activities that won't save your life. Many of our everyday behaviors can be tied back to decreasing the high cortisol levels caused by ongoing stress. For example, sugar is added to many processed foods for a variety of reasons, including that we will eat more of it when stressed. Consuming sugar is an example of a comfort food, because eating sugar reduces cortisol levels so we *feel* less stressed [200]. Yet this habitual suppression of cortisol could reduce our ability to respond appropriately to a serious acute stressor.

Many books could be written detailing the production and secretion of cortisol under different conditions. People disadvantaged by the system, suffering poverty due to social, economic, and political marginalization, or living in a neighborhood where there are high levels of violence tend to have higher levels of cortisol, reflecting their higher stressors and, thus, greater stress hormone levels [201]. People with more advantages and privileges – social, economic, and political – have less stress, and lower levels of cortisol. For example, in the US, Euro-Americans tend to have lower cortisol levels than African Americans [202]. Being a leader in a society may subject one to ever increasing amounts of stress. However, studies show that leaders with a heightened sense of control have lower cortisol levels – a stress-buffering effect. Leadership and ranking higher in society result in such top people having less stress. These persons with power typically cause stress in their subordinates, who, being of lower socioeconomic status, have higher cortisol levels [203].

Studies of British civil servants working in the Whitehall complex of office buildings in London demonstrated that the lower your employment rank, the more stress you suffered and the sicker you became. Personal health-related behaviors of these office workers mattered considerably less. What counted much more was the amount of control they had in their jobs: the lower the control, the more job strain [204].

So, how is cortisol best measured in the body? Cortisol is deposited in the growing scalp-hair shaft. Hair grows about a centimeter a month. By taking lengths of scalp hair and measuring cortisol in centimeter lengths, one learns how much stress the person was under at what time. One study looked at middle-aged men admitted to the hospital with a heart attack and compared their hair cortisol levels over time with those of men admitted for more minor reasons. In the months preceding the hospitalization, those suffering from heart attacks had rising cortisol levels not seen in the others [205]. Cumulative stress often precedes such an unhealthy event.

Cortisol is also increased in a variety of psychiatric disorders and when sleep quality is reduced [206]. Many people report difficulties in sleeping that can be attributed to our stressful societies. When I lived in Nepal where there was no electricity, I never experienced trouble sleeping. A candle or small kerosene lamp provided light, but usually people went to sleep soon after dark. With the availability of various kinds of artificial light, together with much to do after dark, such as shopping, going to movies, and everything at home – especially the electronic devices we binge on – sleep becomes more difficult.

Cortisol rises in late pregnancy, with higher levels found in pregnant women who were abused as children. Adults who have suffered considerable childhood abuse may have blunted responses to stress, in that cortisol levels do not rise as much as in those who did not suffer childhood abuse trauma. Repeated significant stressful events wear out the stress response, so when it is needed to save your life, its effects may not be as robust as they should be. The impacts of early-life abuse on the stress response likely depend on the intensity, duration, and response to the abuse, whose measures are often absent from earlier research reports. Prospective studies, namely enrolling newborns and following them to adulthood, which are needed to better understand the impacts of abuse on stress response, are few. Nevertheless, we know that early-life abuse impacts the adult stress response.

COMMUNITY STRESS. Can we gauge stress levels in a community? During the COVID-19 pandemic, wastewater measurements of SARS-CoV-2 demonstrated the level of this pathogen in a community. Population-level chronic stress levels can be measured by looking at cortisol in wastewater. Such wastewater-based epidemiology may be a better measure than various social surveys that have been conducted on specific individuals or groups gauging their stress levels, because they reflect what is happening in the population. Researchers looking at wastewater at one major US university campus found elevated cortisol levels at the beginning of the semester and during the examination week [207]. Monitoring a variety of wastewater chemicals may provide important windows on what is happening in populations or nations, which is the perspective taken in this book.

SOCIOECONOMIC INEQUALITY AND STRESS

In the US, as the gap between the haves and have-nots, the superrich and the rest of us, has increased massively, trust in government has dropped to an all-time low. Another effect of increased income inequality at the US state level is cardiovascular stress, as measured by laboratory stress tests in which people do mental arithmetic and have to recognize a color word on a computer screen. Those living in more unequal states scored worse on the tests and had less healthy cardiovascular reactivity (changes in blood pressure and pulse) while being tested than those in more equal states [208].

Another experiment exposed a sample of American adults to the cold virus and measured how severe the resulting infection was to understand the immune system. Those participants lower down the socioeconomic ladder caught more colds that were more severe than folks higher up the socioeconomic ladder. Early-life factors were also evident, including, for example, home ownership, a major marker of US socioeconomic and racial discrimination. Not owning a home was a significant persistent stressor, and whether or not their parents owned their own home when the experimental adult subjects were children mattered in catching colds. And the longer the period of home ownership, the less chronic stress for parents, and the less severe their children's colds were years later, as adults [209]. Parental stress is passed on to children via epigenetic means, as discussed below. Too much stress, for too long, or the wrong kind of stress with no relief, assistance, or empathetic witness, is bad for your health and impacts your ability to thwart infections.

TYPES OF STRESS

Not all stress is bad, for it can save your life, as my yak attack story showed. Many of us seek out stress that we find benefits us. I spent many years climbing mountains, and accepted that I could be killed doing so. For years I liked myself best in the mountains. They provided a way of navigating difficult terrain up to mountaintops and then back to their base that made me feel good about myself, despite the risk of dying. Consider this positive stress. Another example I recall is my son Michael fearfully taking his first step with much trepidation, yet after which he beamed delightedly!

In early life, tolerable stress may occur when a close family member is seriously ill or dies, but that stress eventually diminishes if supportive adults help the child. But what happens if there are no supportive adults available to the child? Consider toxic stress as the result of strong, frequent, or prolonged activation of stress response systems in the absence of the buffering protection of a supportive relationship. Toxic stress is ongoing and can't be controlled. It harms the body in ways that cannot be undone later. Toxic stress leading to early-life trauma has major health impacts [210].

What are today's stressors? While few of us will ever face a threatening yak, many people in America must worry about where they will sleep tonight or get their next meal. Others, including the rich, fear being in a mass shooting. The rich worry about being well-off enough. The stressors we are exposed to are not like the yak charge, which was real, but brief. For the most part, today's stressors are psychological and ongoing – chronic stress. Our chronic stress responses, what happens to us when responding to these ongoing tensions, leads to many diseases.

Stanford neuroscientist Robert Sapolsky points out that if you want to avoid stress-related diseases, don't allow yourself to be born poor [206]. Tolerating or even perpetuating a society in which so many people suffer poverty is a political choice, a decision by those in power about who is and who is not entitled to have their basic needs met. For various reasons to be discussed later, the United States' elites have chosen to push policies that produce much poverty in the country. Hence, our high levels of stress, which don't even serve the wealthy.

ELEMENTS OF STRESS BIOLOGY

How do you understand biology? Your parents may not have discussed this when you were a child. In school you likely peered down a microscope and were told those images were cells, or parts within cells. Unless you became a scientist in the realm of biology, most of what you think is true is based on trusting what others you were taught to respect have said or written. Let's dissect concepts of stress at various levels of biology.

TELOMERES. Consider our constituent cells. The heritable material in our genes is DNA. Strands of DNA can unravel, so ends of DNA are capped with telomeres to prevent unraveling. Think of them like the metal or plastic ends of shoelaces. Telomeres shorten over time, and also as a result of long-standing stress. When telomeres become too short, the cell dies. An enzyme, telomerase, can repair the frayed ends. Levels of the enzyme found in the body is a biomarker for this reparative process [211]. With more immiseration, that is oppression and inequity, including social exclusion, political disenfranchisement, and economic deprivation, life is harder. Many studies show that children with more adversity have shorter telomeres. Racialized groups and genders are also associated with different telomere lengths. Telomeres are also shorter in working-class people who have toiled many years at low-pay, high-stress labor. Shorter telomeres and lower levels of the reparative enzyme give another level of bodily evidence of the hardship and suffering undergone by people who are immiserated.

MITOCHONDRIA. Inside the cell are mitochondria. These organelles process food substrates to produce energy the cell needs. Mitochondria have their own genes which come from your mother. They replicate independently of the cell in which they reside in a dynamic process as they divide, fuse, and change shape to satisfy the energy demands of their cell. They are the cell's energy factory. Mitochondria can become defective over time to such an extent that they do not function properly [212]. Many of our chronic diseases stem from mitochondria not working well. Glucose is broken down to energy substrates to power cellular processes. When too much glucose enters the cell and the mitochondria can't keep up with the load, the workshop diverts glucose into fat, which can cause obesity and contribute to diabetes.

MICROBIOME. Much of what we eat is also consumed by our microbiome, namely the trillions of bacteria and other organisms living in our intestine. We feed these microscopic creatures that live within us. Another issue relates to the type of food eaten. A calorie from fructose, a component of table sugar, can change how the liver functions to limit its ability to burn fat. Finally, people's metabolisms differ in their efficiency. A food calorie in is thus not a calorie out. It depends on what form that calorie is in, and whether it feeds your microbiome instead of you. If your food feeds the organisms that live on you, those calories do not go into you. This explains why you can gain weight so easily today with the highly processed, sugar-added, foods we consume.

As a generalization, the less income and resources people have, the less access they have to healthy foods [213]. The mitochondria of people without access to healthy diets also function more poorly. Such mitochondrial dysfunction may explain how dietary factors affect chronic diseases. Chronic stress is more common among people experiencing poverty, which leads to their worse health via these intracellular mechanisms. Epigenetics can help understand how environmental factors, broadly considered, can be transmitted from one generation to another.

EPIGENETICS

It may surprise you to learn that the stress and trauma you experience in your life prior to reproduction can be transmitted to the next generation by nongenomic means – and that the stress and trauma of your ancestors before you may have been passed on to you. This isn't some hocus-pocus theory; it's a biological process known as epigenetics. You began your existence in your maternal grandmother's womb since the ovum that begat you was made there. Your grandmother's circumstances can affect you outside of the DNA in your genes. Aspects of anyone's environment, broadly considered, can affect subsequent generations through epigenetic means. Epigenetic means beyond genetics. One example mentioned above is the increase in oxytocin with positive early-life experiences.

The DNA in your genes codes for producing proteins, the enzymes that make things happen via catalyzing biochemical reactions. There are various ways of regulating this genetic process. Does an enzyme get made or not? How many copies? To understand this process, read the following words: a woman without her man is nothing. Now punctuate that string of words in two ways using standard punctuation marks so the resulting two sentences have polar opposite meanings. A woman, without her man, is nothing. A woman: without her, man is nothing. Consider epigenetics as the punctuation marks for a segment of DNA that expresses a gene in different ways.

Measuring epigenetic markers in the blood may be one way of assessing biological aging to consider ways of changing it [214,215]. Consider them epigenetic clocks [216,217].

Epigenetics explains why conditions affecting a fetus *in utero* can be passed down to that person's children. An example presented earlier was in the Dutch Hunger Winter when children born of mothers without adequate food intake during pregnancy later had diabetes and *their* children had diabetes [27]. Their genes did not change. Epigenetics is one way our DNA seems to be able to respond to the fast-changing world we live in. The field of social epigenomics documents how being lower down in socioeconomic status and being subject to more disadvantage leads to worse health outcomes. Expect progress in this emerging field [218,219]. Meanwhile, stress can wear us out.

ALLOSTASIS AND WEATHERING

Allostasis refers to short-term adaptations to being stressed as a way of maintaining stability. Allostatic load is the term for the body's response to repeated stresses, indicating wear and tear over time that predisposes a person to illness. More common terms might be *stressed* and *stressed out.* Allostatic load has effects on individuals as well as at the neighborhood level and at the macro level where economic and political systems can enhance or diminish the process. National allostatic load might include the various stress-related conditions there such as the high rates of opioid deaths and gun violence. The United States can be considered stressed out.

Individually, allostatic load can be measured by blood pressure and heart rate variability, by blood lipid levels, by how well glucose is metabolized, and by markers of inflammation. Levels of hormones such as adrenaline, vasopressin, cortisol, and oxytocin also factor into these measures. Immiseration of children living in families that must survive under conditions of extreme impoverishment predicts higher adult allostatic load, and, as a result, worse health [220].

Consider international studies. One study looked at Sweden and Lithuania to explain why mortality from heart disease was four times higher in Lithuania than in Sweden. It administered a stress test to 50-year-old men in Vilnius, Lithuania, and compared the results to those of men in Linköping, Sweden. Measures of cortisol, blood pressure, and heart rate showed that Lithuanian men had higher cortisol levels before the stress test and did not mount as big a rise in the chronic stress hormone as those in Sweden [221]. With increasing allostatic load, when the big stressor comes you can't mount as good a response as someone with less load.

A contrasting bodily process to the sympathetic nervous system, which generates the stress response, is the parasympathetic nervous system, which prepares the body to rest and digest rather than to fight or flee. Neurotransmitters carry out this work. One indicator that the parasympathetic system is at work is a small variation in the heartbeat with breathing. This is called heart rate variability. Assuming you have a normal heart, check to see if there are small changes in your pulse while you breathe in and out. Having heart rate variability suggests you aren't that stressed at that time.

Polyvagal theory, a concept developed by Stephen Porges, recognizes that how safe we feel is crucial to our physical and mental health and happiness [222]. The vagus nerve (from Latin, meaning "nerve that wanders") reaches the main organs and both communicates from the organs to the brain and sends messages in the other direction. Polyvagal refers to the multiple functions this nerve has. Feelings of safety and threat are communicated throughout the body via this nerve, which can be considered the conductor of the body's symphony of security and lack thereof. The vagus nerve regulates parasympathetic tone, which is represented by heart rate variability.

We live in a scary world. Whether the fear mongering comes from messages about aliens, invading outsiders, pending economic collapse, or ever-present germs, fear is not a healthy state. Our challenge is to create a safe world. But how safe are we? A *US News and World Report* 2024 ranking of safe countries puts the US 47th out of 89 nations. Few readers would place the United States as the safest nation, and this lack of safety may affect our health through polyvagal mechanisms that reflect whether or not we feel safe.

Constant racial discrimination and racialized violence against African Americans keeps many from ever feeling safe in the US. Arline Geronimus coined the term "weathering" as a process that encompasses the physiological effects on people who live in a racist society where marginalized communities bear the brunt of racial, ethnic, religious, and class discrimination. Understanding weathering is critical to understanding and eliminating population health inequity [202]. Inflammation is the body's process of dealing with weathering and damaged tissue.

SOCIOECONOMIC GRADIENT, STRESS, AND INFLAMMATION

Inflammation, one part of the body's cellular response to irritation or injury, underlies many chronic diseases [223]. A skin abscess or boil is one way the body walls off an acute infection using white blood cells as the inflammatory agent. When the abscess bursts and pus is released, the condition is treated. Chronic (meaning ongoing) cellular inflammatory processes produce atherosclerosis, or narrowing of the arteries supplying the heart muscle. Many different intracellular markers of inflammation can be assessed. To gauge how much chronic inflammation there is in the body, levels of C-reactive protein (CRP) can be measured in blood. Higher CRP levels in the blood indicate more chronic inflammation. Older African Americans have higher CRP levels than older White Americans. This is likely related to the cumulative burden of everyday discrimination over a lifetime, leading to an eternity of higher inflammation [224].

Other sources of stress create inflammation and higher CRP levels. For example, looking at France, Italy, Portugal, Ireland, the UK, Finland, Switzerland, and Australia, we see higher CRP levels among those with less education [225]. In studies of British civil servants doing desk work who were given a stress test, those with lower employment grades had worse outcomes, with higher inflammatory markers. Observing the socio-economic gradient at the cellular level, researchers saw that people ranked lower in work hierarchies had more inflammation.

The socioeconomic gradient discussed above is present at the organ level. Consider the lung. Lung function can easily be assessed by measuring how much air you can blow out forcefully in one second. This indicator is called forced expiratory volume in 1 second (FEV_1). People who are economically immiserated blow out less air than richer folk. A review paper presented the studies demonstrating this around the world [226]. An American study found that people suffering more poverty also have worse lung function than wealthier people. Early-life factors related to being disadvantaged by the system, such as low birthweight, being too lean or too fat, or getting asthma in early life, led to worse lung function as measured by FEV_1 [227]. Having worse lung function sets one up for lung disease with aging [228].

The lung findings are true for the other bodily organs. Once you ask the question about who has healthier organs, the finding is uniform. More impoverished people have worse functioning organs, which sets them up for those organs to become dysfunctional and result in worse health for their owners.

At the individual level, in Chapters 3 and 5, we described how people experiencing poverty and denied resources have more disease and illness as a result of constant multilevel stressors. In Chapter 2 we saw that medical care in the absence of other social investments has less of an impact on improving health in poorer people, independent of the quality of care received. We know that personal behaviors have less impact on these outcomes, as was demonstrated by children from low-income, economically disenfranchised US neighborhoods having worse results after heart transplants than those from richer ones [37]. One reason is that, due to altered biology, impoverished children's bodies have less capacity to accept transplanted hearts. The data across nations show that socioeconomic deprivation matters for many health outcomes, with the United States a prime example. For example, according to the Congressional Budget Office, the richest 1% have over 130 times the income of the bottom 20%. The evidence for the impact of the socioeconomic gradient on health is undeniable.

We began by establishing that socioeconomic deprivation and discrimination create chronic stress in the body, which, in turn, *causes* worse health, by using the same criteria that validated cigarette smoking as being bad for health in the 1964 US Surgeon General's report [192]. Few people smoke cigarettes in the United States today. Those who do are mostly poor, as smoking relieves their stress, which is common for most people in America, but especially for those living in poverty. Consider stress as the twenty-first-century tobacco.

One further issue to explore is obesity. Doing so will help integrate many ideas presented so far.

OBESITY AND STRESS

The United States is among the most obese nations [229]. A variety of conditions act synergistically to make us fatter than people in other countries. Body mass index (BMI) is a common calculation dividing one's weight (in kilograms) by height (in meters) squared (kg/m^2). Consider normal as 18 to 25. Above that is overweight and above 30 labels one as obese. Despite BMI being a flawed measure, as it doesn't distinguish fat tissue from muscle (that is, a very muscular person could have the same BMI as one with little muscle), it allows for comparisons across countries. How does the US rank for adults among nations using this measure for obesity? The Global Obesity Observatory puts the US 10th for women [230]. All the countries with more obese people are small islands in the Pacific such as Nauru, Samoa, and Tahiti, likely for reasons related to the impact of colonization on land, people, and cultures, including foodways, and the resulting sedentary lifestyle and processed imported foods [231]. Why this global distribution?

Recalling my youth, almost no people looked significantly overweight in either the United States or Canada. Our family ate meals prepared by my mother at home, and we almost never ate at a restaurant. In 1969

I spent a year in Nepal. Of the people I encountered, I can remember only one woman whom one might consider overweight just based on visual information. She was the wife of a wealthy man. There were princesses in the Nepalese Royal Family who might also have been either overweight or obese, but I know this only from pictures. People said that you had to be rich to be overweight. That meant you didn't have much of any physical work to do and had access to plenty of food. Working as a doctor in a community health project a week's walk from the road in western Nepal in the 1970s, and a decade later setting up a remote teaching hospital for Nepali doctors in far west Nepal, I did not recall encountering overweight people. There was also no advertising of any kind there. No restaurants except in Kathmandu, the capital city, and those were mostly patronized by tourists. When I offered to take a Nepali family to a restaurant, they didn't understand why they should go. Along major trails where porters carried goods, there were makeshift inns for them to sleep and eat – mostly food that they carried and prepared themselves. Otherwise, everyone ate an, as yet, uncolonized diet and did intensive physical labor.

When I was back in the United States in the 1980s, encounters with the people who were clinically obese became common. The presence of obese people varied across the country. The highest concentration I personally encountered was as a keynote speaker at a 2012 public health conference in West Virginia. Many of these state, county, and local officials were obese. They worked in public health. It made me think about what might cause this contradiction, as it seemed to be to me.

Consider your own experiences regarding obesity and what you can infer from them. You may suffer from this common condition. Today there is more acceptance of different weights and pressure to end discrimination based on weight – or sizeism – in society. Considerable stigma still exists, reinforced by a large weight-loss industry.

There is also the controversial perspective that obesity is not a disease, that you can have health at every size, suggesting you can have metabolically healthy obesity – meaning having a BMI over 29, but without having increased risks of heart disease and death. Some estimates suggest that perhaps 20% of obese Americans are metabolically healthy. But there is no consensus on what being metabolically healthy means, nor agreement on whether it actually exists. Part of the reason is that being called metabolically healthy requires estimating various clinical parameters, typically at one point in time. There are no long-term cohort studies following such people to see whether or not they eventually experience obesity-related disease. The jury is out on whether metabolically healthy obesity really exists or is a transient concept [232]. The last word on obesity will be far into the future.

We've already talked about stress that your mother may have faced when you were in the womb that can lead to your being overweight. Being born of low birthweight followed by rapid catch-up growth, experiencing toxic stress, and being abused in early life also make you more likely to be overweight or obese. Many studies substantiate that physical and sexual abuse of girls leads to overeating and obesity [233]. The adverse childhood experiences (ACEs) studies described in Chapter 4 provide other examples.

People in the United States report some of the highest stress levels in the world. How do we cope with our stress and the social pain that stress causes? Among the ways we cope is through opioids. Recall we consume over three-quarters of the world's supply. Another way to cope is to eat comfort foods. Foods high in fat, sugar, and salt inhibit the release of cortisol, our chronic stress hormone. Loneliness, now common, is assuaged by eating food.

Using food as self-medication for emotional stress is linked to the way that food economics has changed drastically over the past 75 years. Food used to be expensive and of relatively low caloric density, and it took time to prepare meals. Food was eaten together at home during typical mealtimes, a few times a day (typically two in Nepal, three here in the US where affordable). A century ago, most working people in the US had a great deal of physical work to do that required caloric fuel, so a healthy appetite was imperative. That is how we were programmed to survive then.

Fast forward to the present. Food is incredibly cheap, is highly processed with high caloric density, can be prepared in minutes, and tends to be eaten alone around the clock. We have been programmed to eat a great deal to do our work. But automation has removed the physical work and many of us are mouse workers. We drag a so-called rodent across a pad. That doesn't require many calories. We eat large amounts and often become overweight and obese. Consider this the nutrition transition [234].

Recall the epidemiological transition from diseases of young bowels to diseases of old arteries discussed in Chapter 2. The nutrition transition took us from low-calorie, less processed foods requiring time to prepare and eaten at mealtimes with others to high-calorie, ultra-processed, fatty, sweet, and salty foods eaten alone almost continuously. Note how many fast-food businesses are open for long hours to supply our desires, or, some say, to feed the addictions they benefit from. Think of all the products (small-sized bags of foods we crave) that allow us to constantly snack – the equivalent of grazing for cattle.

The situation is not so uniform around the country or the world. Unlike my initial experiences in Nepal, where the rich were overweight, now economically marginalized people are more likely to be overweight. Almost everywhere you look, thinner people tend to be richer and less likely to eat ultra-processed food. Once, while dining while in Washington, DC, I asked what characterized expensive restaurants there. The answer was, "Small portions." The socioeconomic gradient is at work. Across and within countries, greater income inequality is correlated with higher rates of obesity. In societies with bigger income gaps, lower-income people are more likely to be more stressed, have less access to healthy foods, and experience more behavioral injustice, including little time and place to safely exercise. As a result, more obesity is present.

What about the new expensive weight-loss injectable drug semaglutide that has commanded so much media attention? It was developed to treat diabetes, likely needs to be taken for a lifetime, and has limited benefits. Semaglutide, and other GLP-1 blockbusters, represent an anti-obesity gold rush that is typical of modern drugs, namely they maintain people with chronic conditions. They provide a very profitable revenue stream for the weight-loss industry that won't let obesity or their income streams melt or wither away.

Obesity is a complex problem that is related to the physiological and social effects of stress in our society, along with the commercialization of one important segment of the stress-relief industry, namely – marketing ultra-processed foods. Our food industry needs to grow to continue generating profits, but our population is not increasing much. The way for the corporations to prosper is to get us to eat more through irresistible food advertising.

Thus, our social world shapes our biology, as we adapt our lives to our stress and consumer-driven environments. Therefore, we must next address how we convert food into energy.

METABOLIC SYNDROME

As type 2 diabetes, hypertension, lipid disorders, and obesity are increasing around the world, the term metabolic syndrome is used to describe the clustering of these risk factors or conditions that can lead to heart disease, diabetes, and stroke. While it has no commonly agreed definition, elevated blood pressure, bigger waistlines, harmful fatty substances in blood, and the inability to process glucose are essential features of metabolic syndrome. Metabolic syndrome is the inappropriate storage of energy in the wrong form in cells that shouldn't store it. Metabolic syndrome affects younger and younger people. Insulin resistance is a prime metabolic defect, namely the presence of high levels of this hormone circulating in the blood and that doesn't function properly to lower glucose. Poorly functioning mitochondria are likely the harbinger of metabolic syndrome. Inflammation is also at work.

Prenatal stress, together with low birthweight, predispose the body to this condition. Fetal development shows signs of being affected by conditions outside the uterus, for example maternal stress, which alters fetal physiology in ways that might have some long-term benefits for viability – survival to adulthood to enable reproduction [232]. When prenatal conditions are harsh, namely that the period outside the womb will produce challenges to limit long-term survival, fetal organ development may speed up. This can result in premature birth, with increased risk of having compromised organs and being of low birthweight. Examples were given in Chapter 4 of such fetal growth malleability during periods of environmental stress, including natural experiments such as the nutritional stress of the Dutch Hunger Winter, the various psychosocial stresses associated with the 9/11 collapse of the World Trade Center towers, Hurricane Katrina, and the 2016 US presidential election. In early gestation the heart is being formed, in mid-gestation the lung and kidneys, and in late gestation fat tissue. The various metabolic consequences of inadequate development *in utero* may comprise metabolic syndrome. Preconception stress also contributes to this through the epigenetic and other modifications described previously.

Chronic stress, measured by the levels of cortisol in hair in populations, together with low social support, was linked to a higher prevalence of metabolic syndrome in one Lithuanian study where those with higher levels of cortisol in their hair and lack of social support had more signs of metabolic syndrome [235].

Some US studies suggest only one in eight adults may have a healthy metabolism [236]. ACEs and early-life trauma are implicated. Nutrition and dietary factors are also at work here. Sugar, a ubiquitous food additive, is used by the ultra-processed food industry, along with so many other ingredients. When I spent a year in Nepal, sugar was absent in traditional Nepali diets. There was very little tooth decay, as evidenced in a countrywide dental survey, despite there being no flossing or brushing. After returning to the US in 1970, I was shocked to read about how breakfast cereal manufacturers were adding sugar to their product so it would taste better and help get your child to eat his or her cereal. The skillful American advertising campaigns were mouthwatering. There were congressional hearings about the process of providing empty calories in most cereal brands. Harvard's chair of its Department of Nutrition testified for the cereal industry. Even today academics who should know better are bought off to serve corporate interests, using their academic status to make lies seem like facts. Mistakenly, I thought this practice would be stopped. How wrong I was.

Life is uncertain; eat dessert first! Given how sweet so many products are, it is almost like we are eating dessert all day long. Sugar is everywhere! Many, if not most, breakfast cereals today are close to half sugar. Almost a teaspoon of sugar is added to hamburger buns at McDonald's, supposedly to help feed the yeast. Refined sugar is almost impossible to avoid. Is that the real problem? Remember, desserts spelled backwards is stressed. The real problem is the chronic stress we face constantly.

Pediatric endocrinologist Robert Lustig spells out much of the complicated science about metabolic syndrome in great detail [212]. He expounds on the "a calorie in is not a calorie out" concept mentioned earlier, which is certainly not universally accepted. A different perspective to the dietary guidelines he discussed reflects the key message of this book. Don't be poor, or have poor parents. Be born where there is less inequality and have a supportive early life. These are not individual choices, but are population-level effects of how resources and entitlement to resources are distributed, which are choices made by a society.

The challenge is to reduce chronic stress in society. Reserve the stress response to keeping us safe from danger or an immediate threat, as it was designed to do. Then we won't need comfort foods. Then we can all have a greater chance at a long and healthy life.

BIOLOGY OF AGING

Given that most of us would rather live a longer life and age gracefully, what can we say about the biology of successful aging? It is easy to say that we want our mitochondria to be healthy and limit the ends of our DNA becoming shorter. We also want to have less inflammation and to sidestep weathering [237]. There won't be a pill for these issues, nor a surgical procedure to correct organ failures. We need to level the steep socioeconomic gradient – inequality and inequity. That will require changes in the social, economic, and political structures of our society. We need a social revolution. That prescription needs to become a part of our mental makeup.

That brings us to mental health. Is America driving us crazy?

CHAPTER SEVEN

Is America Driving You Crazy?

What you need is a gramme of soma. All the advantages of Christianity and alcohol; none of their defects. … People are happy; they get what they want, and they never want what they can't get. And if anything should go wrong, there's soma.

Aldous Huxley, *Brave New World*

We have argued that rather than looking at an individual's health and the diseases they have, we must look at the country or population in which that individual resides. That is because factors outside of a person's control are the primary determinants of his or her health. Two issues matter: the amount of economic inequality in that society or country, and how advantageous the circumstances are there to nurture the child in the first 1,000 days after conception. Those are not under the control of the individual or parent, but depend on the social and political environment in that population or country. We have looked at a variety of illnesses and disease conditions to show that living in the United States may be bad for your health. Mental health is no different. We begin with an actual grand rounds presentation in the psychiatry department at the University of Washington and then go on to see how the US does in mental health comparisons across nations.

The 2004 World Health Organization (WHO) World Mental Health Survey found considerably more mental illness in the US than in other examined countries [238]. I teamed up with University of Washington psychiatrist Dr. Paul Ciechanowski to do a grand rounds in that department the same year. In grand rounds, which are regular events for doctors in American hospitals, doctors typically meet and learn about a patient, exploring features of their case and treatment, and presenting an overview of the illness.

Paul and I presented the patient we called, "Emma Erika." He and I discussed this patient's mental health issues. Emma Erika was actually our pseudonym for the country America. This was a major deviation from the usual patient described, who was always an individual person with various mental problems. Instead we showed that the country had much mental illness. We based this on the 2004 WHO study just published. We pointed out that this patient was not very healthy overall. A key reason presented for her poor health was her income inequality – a characteristic of a population, not an individual. Paul and I concluded that social or societal medicine was the treatment needed for this patient's illness, that is, medicine affecting the social determinants of health we met earlier, in Chapters 2 and 3. A "medicine" to treat a population, in this case the United States of America, may be different from the medicine to treat individuals. Although some may say that, to treat US mental illness, perhaps many people in the USA should be taking a psychiatric medicine. Instead we were asking psychiatrists to think about a country as the "patient" that requires a different response.

MENTAL ILLNESS IN THE USA AND OTHER NATIONS

Let's dissect the World Mental Health surveys that led to the psychiatry grand rounds [238]. The countries surveyed were Belgium, China (Beijing and Shanghai), Colombia, France, Germany, Italy, Japan, Lebanon, Mexico, the Netherlands, Nigeria, Spain, Ukraine, and the United States. Face-to-face household surveys of over 60,000 adults were done in those countries between 2001 and 2003. The mental illness conditions they focused on were related to anxiety, mood, impulse control, and substance use, and classified as serious or not. The 12-month prevalence of these combined conditions showed the US as having 26.4% of the population in one of those categories, which was the highest score. A total of 7.7% were classified as serious, which was again the highest grouping. Of the four conditions, the US had the highest rate of each except for substance use, which was higher only in Ukraine. The US also provided the most treatment available, which suggests treating these conditions has limited effect. That study has been referenced over 4,400 times, which means it has been taken seriously. But it is only one piece of evidence.

There have been other similar attempts with consistent findings, namely that mental illnesses are common, they begin in childhood, and they have strong adverse effects in adulthood [239]. Once again, the US is the leader. Harvard's Professor Ronald Kessler has been a major force in pursuing these kinds of investigations. He ranks among the most cited researchers in the world. A different perspective uses the disability-adjusted life years (DALYs) measure from the Institute for Health Metrics and Evaluation. In its 2019 evaluation, the United States also had the most mental illnesses.

Harvard University has a center – The World Mental Health Survey Initiative – that uses a structured diagnostic interview to obtain cross-national information. It has a huge list of publications on its website. Many of them are specific to a single disorder and region of the world. So far it has produced six volumes in a series of WHO World Mental Health Surveys. Perhaps it makes sense that the country with the most mental illness in the world, the USA, also produces the most reports.

I added a class on mental health in my population health courses at the University of Washington, where I posed these questions to my class: "What are the signs and symptoms Emma Erika presents, what is her diagnosis, and what treatment shall we prescribe?" Students have previously done an exercise called a Population Health Web Ramble where, using sources on the internet and questions they must address, they discover for themselves the less than stellar health outcomes of the United States, presented in this book's earlier chapters. Equipped with this method they soon discover the WHO study and subsequent ones that confirm the substantial mental illness issues in America. Many students who have themselves been diagnosed with various mental illnesses are reassured to discover they are not alone.

We have to face a troubling finding. Mental illness is a serious problem in the United States. What actually is mental illness?

MENTAL HEALTH. Mental health is a necessary component of our overall health. The term *mental health* has multiple meanings and implications, together with associated controversies. The Centers for Disease Control and Prevention (CDC) glosses it by saying, "Mental health includes our emotional, psychological, and social well-being. It affects how we think, feel, and act. It also helps determine how we handle stress, relate to others, and make healthy choices." This is reminiscent of the WHO's 1948 definition of health as, "a state of complete physical, mental, and social well-being and not merely the absence of disease or infirmity." The WHO definition, easily remembered, has stood the test of time and can be applied universally.

Mental illness will affect many, if not most, people at some point over their life course in the US. The stigma surrounding mental illness may be decreasing as more and more people are acknowledging their mental problems. Is mental illness increasing? Why does living in the United States contribute to worse mental health in people there? There now exists a a *Lancet Psychiatry* Commission on youth mental health to explore the crisis [240], as increasing trends are seen in different parts of the world.

Just as other health disorders are linked to inequality, there is a strong relationship linking mental illness to income inequality. This can also be seen for depression, anxiety, and schizophrenia, among others. We have higher rates of each of these disorders among US states, with higher rates in more income-unequal states. Inequality is bad not just for our physical health, but for our mental health.

MENTAL HEALTH DRUG USE AND HIERARCHY

We have highlighted the importance of economic inequality and early-life issues for several health and illness concerns that are themselves political issues. What are some mental health implications of those ideas? Let's begin by looking at drugs of abuse, specifically cocaine and opioids. Over three-quarters of the world's opioids are consumed in the US, making this a serious concern.

One study looked at monkeys who form a status ordering when housed in social groups. These groups comprise an alpha monkey, a beta monkey, a gamma monkey, and so on. After establishing their hierarchy, the monkeys had a catheter implanted to allow them to self-administer cocaine. The dominant monkey did not use much cocaine, whereas there was increasing use in those lower down the ranking. Cocaine gives the user feelings of power that may blunt the stressful experience of being of lower status. Cocaine binds to dopamine transporters, enhancing the impact of dopamine. Dopamine affects the brain's reward system and is the driver of pleasure and motivation. The dominant monkey has enough reward and pleasure from being the top simian and doesn't need cocaine [241]. Another study looked at isolated rats versus those who lived with others. Those who were on their own consumed large quantities of morphine that was offered, while those who lived with others did not seem to need it [242]. Results of nonhuman animal studies should not imply that there must be similar findings in humans. But they can guide understanding of what is observed in our species. These animal studies suggest that people under great stressors, and here we must include living in poverty, having a mental illness, being unhoused or trafficked, as well as those suffering from isolation or loneliness, may also seek comfort or self-medication in drug use that can become a substance use disorder.

Implications for human societies follow. Drug use among countries is related to income inequality. The United States stands out with both high inequality and high drug use [161]. Rates of opioid deaths in the United States are higher than elsewhere. Users tend to be people who are socially and/or economically disenfranchised. But even the well-off have problems. Adults who had early-life adverse childhood experiences (ACEs) are more likely to inject drugs and/or be medicated by their physicians with psychotropic drugs. It is a vicious cycle: more early-life adversity, that is, a compromised early life, can lead to self-medication through drug or alcohol use and frequently also physician medication, rather than psychological support through therapy in a broken and managed healthcare system. This can create conditions under which the next generation may also have to face early-life adversity.

HAPPINESS AND PLEASURE

We humans engage in a range of behaviors to get dopamine hits, including through psychoactive drug use. More inequality is associated with more drug use.

Dopamine is involved in both our feeling pleasure and our feeling pain [243]. Human dopamine transmission occurs with chocolate, sex, nicotine, drugs such as cocaine and methamphetamine, and a host of other stimuli that include eating good food, listening to music, and having social interactions. Dopamine release produces pleasure, but with diminishing returns as more is released. The next piece of chocolate never tastes as good as the first. Similarly for shopping, gaming, and pornography. We sometimes feel the pleasure of buying stuff, but don't even open the package when it arrives. The body tries to seek a balance so there is not too much pleasure, just like for stress. Too much chronic stress is bad for us. Altering the balance can result in a huge stress load, being stressed out, which weighs us down and does us in. People under chronic stress seek relief by seeking more pleasure. As they do so, cortisol, the chronic stress hormone, helps the brain release more dopamine to make them *seek* even more pleasure, which becomes elusive. We *can* have too much of a good thing.

What balances the pleasure so we don't have too much? The opposite of pleasure can be worry, anxiety, pain, boredom, and generally not feeling good. Pain can be thought of as the opposite of pleasure. The centers for pleasure and pain reside close together in the brain.

Too much pleasure increases our brain's tolerance to the stimulus that used to give us pleasure. We need more and more of it to feel good. The US drug industry's push to get doctors to prescribe more opioids to deal with our increasing pain didn't help. With that source now diminished, people turn to other reservoirs of opioids that are easier to access in America, such as heroin and fentanyl, especially the latter. As someone uses more opioids for pain, the pain no longer diminishes, but may become worse, because the brain has reset the pleasure–pain balance in the direction of more pain. That can lead to self-harm.

One way someone may cope with mental anguish and emotional distress is to replace that feeling with a painful stimulus. Nonsuicidal self-injury, such as cutting one's forearm or thigh, is one way some people try to cope with much less tolerable distress and severe emotions. In the emergency department I sometimes saw words like "ugly" inscribed on a thigh to help grapple with those feelings. Such incisions helped one manage – a form of psychic regulation. Self-harm is increasingly common today and not limited to the United States. ACEs and early-life adversity amplify such psychological and physical pain.

Could our increasing pain be a response to the many forms of indulgence or luxury that have become normalized? Consider the mobile phone and the smartwatch which so many now own, but which no longer give them much pleasure. The smartphone is today's digital dopamine delivery device. We live in a world that is saturated with dopamine, but we can never get enough. Being able to access social media can give us pleasure, but that pleasure is soon replaced with pain and anxiety as we make status comparisons. The more behaviors we engage in to release more dopamine, paradoxically, the less dopamine we have to make us feel good.

In Chapter 1 we discussed the pressure to be happy. This pressure is so great that we have medicalized ordinary unhappiness as a psychiatric problem requiring medication. Even cancer patients are encouraged to "be positive" while undergoing grueling treatments, dealing with the loss of body parts, and facing potential death. Yet for all the pressure on us to be happy, as pointed out in Chapter 1, happiness in the US has been steadily declining. That state of contentment we're expected to embrace is escaping us. Recall that the United States Declaration of Independence gave us the right to pursue happiness, not necessarily to attain it.

Happiness differs from pleasure in that pleasure is momentary, while happiness reflects long-term contentment. Happiness does not come from the pursuit of pleasure which is synonymous with reward. The more pleasure you seek, the less happy you will become, given the increasing tolerance to dopamine. Unlike dopamine, the neurotransmitter serotonin is associated with happiness. When serotonin is released, you say, "This feels good. I don't need anymore." Serotonin is a mood stabilizer.

Depression can be understood as the lack of sufficient serotonin released between synaptic junctions. There are many varieties of depression, so let's consider milder forms that reflect low mood. So-called selective serotonin reuptake inhibitors (SSRIs) are drugs that increase serotonin between synaptic junctions in the brain, to be taken up by the next neuron inline as chemical messengers. These antidepressant drugs are heavily marketed to us and are often prescribed with little to no effort to find out whether someone's depression is situational – caused by a recent event or circumstances – or chronic. Many people feel that if they are not "happy," they must be depressed.

These neurotransmitters, dopamine and serotonin, first identified in the 1950s, have become a modern scientific way of looking at pleasure, pain, and happiness. But the concepts of happiness, pain, and pleasure are as old as humanity. Modern science is not necessary to understand these human characteristics.

And as all conditions we've looked at thus far, early-life conditions affect how cells in the brain communicate with one another and impact happiness, pain, and pleasure. Those who, in early life, have been subjected to trauma or ACEs, are more likely to use illicit drugs and seek pleasure in ways that can be self-destructive. The same is true for forms of insecure attachment, which have been previously discussed in the early life and biology chapters (Chapters 4 and 6). Early life matters. Comparing the US with other nations, we have substantial populations with ACEs and insecure attachment [244].

STRESS DURING PREGNANCY

A pregnant person who is suffering chronic stress sends hormonal signals through the placental wall that cause adjustments in fetal development. Chronic stress in the first third of a pregnancy leads to greater risk of many forms of mental illness in some children, as found in the Dutch Hunger Winter. Other studies show that stress during pregnancy is associated with later child depression [245], as is being born of low birthweight. Schizophrenia is more likely to develop in a person whose pregnant parent experienced chronic stress in the second month of pregnancy [246]. Chronic stress during weeks 12–21 of gestation is associated with the development of attention deficit hyperactivity disorder (ADHD) [247]. None of these are absolutes. They are patterns that have been observed of associations between being born to a chronically stressed parent and having an increased risk of suffering from such mental illnesses.

SOCIAL PSYCHIATRY

My 1972 medical school rotation in an inpatient psychiatry ward was set up as a therapeutic community. The patients and the doctors all met in a large room and had long discussions together. At that time, mental illness treatment was accepted as socially based. Drugs were used to treat some mental illness conditions, but were limited because of significant side effects. Social or community psychiatry was at work [248]. It wasn't to last, however, as the pharmacological treatment of mental health problems became dominant.

Today the idea of involving a community to treat mental issues is mostly gone in Western biomedical settings, but with one long-standing example remaining that is presented below. Community psychiatry and mental health now refer to treatment outside of a hospital, the repair shop model, and not to the mental illness problem residing at the community level. We have been inundated with the new concept that mental illness results from a chemical imbalance in the brain. Just what is this "chemical imbalance?"

CHEMICAL IMBALANCE IN THE BRAIN

With the marketing of Prozac® in 1986, the concept of mental illness as due to a biochemical imbalance in the brain began. Prozac® (fluoxetine) is an SSRI specifically marketed for depression. The successful advertising campaign led to most people's perception today that these chemical imbalances are the root cause of mental illness. Hence the growth of biological psychiatry or biopsychiatry, meaning mental illness has predominantly biological roots. Biopsychiatry treats mental health problems through a psychopharmaceutical approach, which is how most psychiatrists in the United States now practice. They mostly prescribe drugs and vary regimens, but rarely practice psychotherapy anymore. There is no time for that in the 15-minute appointment period allotted as reimbursable in managed care regimens. Some psychiatrists have changed their practices to self-pay in order to have time for psychotherapy. Almost half of psychiatrists do not accept commercial healthcare insurance [249]. Many patients seek counseling outside of psychiatrists' offices if they can pay.

Who gets to see a psychiatrist or other mental health practitioner in the US? It is unlikely to be a person with little or no income, someone on Medicaid, or someone otherwise unable to self-pay. Medicaid provides limited psychiatric hospitalization in many states, with tenfold variation in length of stay amongst them. Given that the socioeconomic gradient is at work with mental illness, those most in need, those with the least access to basic resources all around, are less likely to get attention, except, as we shall see, in prison.

Unfortunately, the entire concept of a chemical imbalance as a cause of mental illness is an urban legend [250]. While there are varying levels of neurotransmitters in the brain that may impact mental health, much more is going on [251]. We want a simple explanation for mental illness, and this one is easy to accept, given the availability of drugs to supposedly restore the "chemical balance." This easy fix has less social stigma, because it suggests there is something wrong physically, rather than cognitively or emotionally or related to the political aspects of living in the United States. Contradictory findings that challenge that simple perspective may be rejected – by both patients (who often want the quick fix with minimal introspection or work) and many psychiatrists (who want the billable hours with minimal analysis or work). We can't cling to the chemical imbalance meme. There is more at stake.

Attention is being paid to neuroplasticity, which looks at adaptive and structural changes in the brain. Brain neurons can alter their communications with one another. Brain plasticity helps explain recovery from strokes and traumatic brain injury. Myriad environmental factors, including stress, psychological trauma, and sociocultural factors, influence the brain's wiring. Brain imaging studies help localize areas of concern. Such a brain-centered approach to treating mental illness is in early stages. Cognitive behavioral therapy (CBT) is one effective neuroplastic treatment. Expect therapeutic progress here.

I was taught that schizophrenia, a serious chronic mental illness affecting cognition, had the same prevalence around the world, and that lifelong drug treatment was required. Later studies showed varying rates of the condition worldwide, however, with high rates in North America and Europe. This variation is due in part to the fact that there is no consensus in how schizophrenia is diagnosed, viewed, and treated globally today [252], and perhaps also in part due to the fact that, because there is a profitable temporary fix in pharmaceutical prescriptions, the diagnosis may be more frequently given. Other mental illness categories follow similar variations.

Today, in a few rich countries, schizophrenia may be considered a temporary condition, sometimes treated by addressing family and community dynamics. For centuries, in Gheel (now Geel), Belgium, people with major psychiatric illness, such as schizophrenia, were put in family foster care homes instead of hospitals. This is one of the oldest examples of treating psychiatric conditions without medicines. Today, by focusing not on rules to follow but on what an individual "patient" and their carer(s) do in seeking understanding and acceptance, they do very well there without drugs. Some call this a careBnB [249]. There has been considerable media publicity generated with hopes to emulate this elsewhere, but what is typically missing is a community tradition. The workshop model of using drugs remains the major focus in most places. In the United States, schizophrenia is still treated almost universally with antipsychotic medications, some of which have severe side effects, such as tardive dyskinesia – involuntary movements of the limbs and tongue, which can make the person appear even more mentally ill. The newer atypical antipsychotics have fewer side effects. In prisons, where many with serious mental illness are housed, they may get drug treatment, but rarely supportive psychotherapy or other wraparound services.

In the United States, we treat schizophrenics as potentially dangerous social pariahs to be locked away or kept out of public sight. But people who here might be diagnosed as schizophrenic, or as having schizotypal disorder, may be considered shamans or specialist healers in other parts of the world. My experiences with such healers in Nepal has been confirmed by reputable scholars who present evidence that this phenomenon is not uncommon [253]. By perceiving schizophrenia as an eccentricity that, in some circumstances, might be beneficial to society, rather than as a tragic mental disease to be medicated into numbness, those living with this condition have a place in society, which minimizes the impact of their illness. So, what constitutes a mental illness?

MENTAL ILLNESS AND TREATMENTS

What is deemed a mental illness has changed considerably over time and has also varied between places. In 1952 the American Psychiatric Association produced the *Diagnostic and Statistical Manual of Mental Disorders* (DSM for short) to classify mental conditions to have a common language based on signs and symptoms. At that time the DSM recognized 106 mental illnesses. Some of these illness classifications, such as homosexuality, have been removed in subsequent editions while many others have been added. The original DSM was a slim volume, whereas the 2022 DSM-5-TR edition is daunting at almost 2,000 pages [254]. Yet the manual has become indispensable in mental health care because, in order for insurance to cover any treatment in the US, there must be a diagnostic code from the DSM. The DSM, translated into many languages, has thus become the world standard for mental illness care, and is the basis for the mental illness sections of the *International Classification of Diseases* (ICD). Documentation for all medical care delivered increasingly uses a form of such diagnostic coding.

Mental illness diagnoses remain based on symptoms. To be given a diagnosis requires the presence of a certain number of symptoms from a list of potential ones. Two people with the same DSM diagnosis could have met the criteria despite presenting mostly different symptoms. The treatments are also based on symptom relief. It is like treating chest pain from a heart attack with pain medicine, and not fixing the damaged heart. This treatment may make it easier for the physician to send the patient home, but it may not resolve the patient's illness. Of course much of the practice of medicine deals with symptom relief. Although patients may benefit, we argue that more is needed, namely treating the population.

Despite the popularity of the biopsychiatric approach (namely mental illness results from a chemical imbalance in the brain that requires drug treatment) to understanding and treating mental health concerns, the pathological or anatomic basis for most mental illness is unknown today, despite earlier experiments to modify the brains of the mentally ill. Such a statement comes from Thomas Insel who, for years, was the director of the National Institute of Mental Health [249].

Consider the frontal lobes, our social organ. In order for us to make sense of, and respond to, social cues, our frontal lobes must be connected to the rest of our brain. The history of treating mental illness includes many barbaric practices, such as lobotomy, which severs the frontal lobe connections from the rest of the brain. Its inventor received the Nobel Prize in Medicine in 1949. Lobotomies were popular throughout the 1950s and were used to treat a range of psychosocial disorders, from rebellious personalities to psychosis. President John F Kennedy's sister had this surgery, which left her in a vegetative state. Fortunately, lobotomies are no longer performed, yet some might consider psychotropic medication practices as the modern-day form of lobotomy. Consider how we provide drugs that affect the brain to children and teens, as long as they have healthcare insurance, who complain of struggles just keeping up with daily life. Given that the United States consumes about half of all the drugs used to treat mental illness in the world, will we eventually recognize the dangers of overmedicating emotional and mental health concerns? Given the possibility of SSRI drugs increasing violent behavior, we should err on the side of caution. This is not to say these drugs don't have any value; however, we have to look at the big picture of mental illness in the US.

Psychiatric treatments depend on one's teaching and experience. These treatments vary greatly around the world. Yet American views on mental illness have affected other countries due to the ICD classifications on mental illness, and the DSM. They have been disproportionately determined by American researchers together with successful marketing. Americanized ways of treating mental illness supplant local perspectives around the world [255]. Cross-cultural psychiatry, the concept that mental illness has different conceptualizations in different cultures, contrasts with the biomedical perspective that disease is invariant around the world. Western biopsychiatry treatment concepts have prevailed to a large degree. Given that the US has so much mental illness, it may not be in another country's best interest to adopt American perspectives. Suppose you wanted to hire a plumber to do work for your house. One presented the most expensive bid. You investigated by going to that person's house and discovered he lived in a stinking cesspool. Would you hire that plumber?

Our near-universal embrace of biopsychiatry and the notion of "better living through chemistry" have led to an unfocused view of mental health and illness. With a poor understanding of the biological basis of mental illnesses, we have a troubled view of how to treat them. We know much about the brain and how our brains influence our cognition, behaviors, emotions, and impulses. We prefer quick-fix psychiatric medications. We've missed understanding how our environment – the external effects of living in the modern world – impacts our mental state.

Are there other explanations to consider?

US MENTAL ILLNESS

Living in the United States today means surviving in a society where the social fabric has been ravaged. The current mental health crisis is really a political crisis with mental health effects. This crisis will not be treated with more mental illness services. Teletherapy or telepsychiatry has become common. Is such virtual care effective? While some individuals attest to its value, virtual care or other forms of psychotherapy are unlikely to resolve the country's problem. Surely you ask, isn't some care better than none? The very costly US mental illness therapy industry lacks expert consensus that much of it is effective. I'm not advocating for no care for mental illness, just as I'm not against care for various illnesses and diseases people have (I get medical treatment), it is just that a stronger population or political medicine must *also* be given. The political crisis underpinning our mental illnesses must be addressed. This begins in the next chapter. But first, more detail on the circumstances producing the problem.

Living in the United States today can be compared to our being lobotomized through the profound and rapid technological transformation of our society. Communities, our social organs, have been cast adrift as we are more and more alone together. Increasing isolation, exacerbated by the COVID-19 pandemic and enhanced by individualized responses, has created destabilizing chronic stress. We eat alone, travel alone, work alone, and limit contact with other human beings to the virtual realm. We are addicted to social media to connect us to others, yet digital media further isolates us from interacting face to face. Pets, such as dogs and cats, are our companions today. While those exploited and dehumanized in our socioeconomic hierarchy are more affected, none of us is spared this stress. We need to go on a digital diet. The most effective response is not more treatment for mental illness, but working for a societal transformation to be less stressed.

And as mental health problems have grown recently, suicides in the United States have been rising, especially among those aged 10–24. Socioeconomic factors can lead to suicidal behavior, as do easy access to guns, online bullying, and social comparisons, together with media coverage that can lead others to copy the behavior. We've also discussed suicide as one of the deaths of despair among middle-aged White peoples and others. State-level income inequality determines suicide mortality rates. Writing on suicide in 1897, Émile Durkheim, one of the founders of sociology, said, "suicide varies inversely with degree of integration of the social groups of which the individual forms a part." With more inequality breeding more isolation, this perspective remains unchallenged today.

Consider teenagers' issues today. When he proposed his stages of psychosocial development, psychoanalyst Erik Erikson theorized that adolescents need an identity. Today, however, the iGeneration, or Gen Z (those born between 1995 and 2012), is adrift and lacking any security, roots, and anchors. Teenagers today are confused regarding their self-esteem and well-being, while being unprepared for an adulthood that is increasingly unaffordable [256].

Mental illness on US college campuses is surging, with a large demand for treatment, and rates of anxiety and depression are at historically high levels. Smartphone-based childhood has supplanted play-based childhood and resulted in much anxiety [257]. Student suicides are increasing, with attendant challenges and consternation for faculty and administrators.

Increasingly, caregivers who cannot deal with the behaviors of their adolescent charges bring them to emergency departments seeking help, a new phenomenon I didn't experience as an emergency physician. Caretakers, who now cannot deal with their children's behaviors, often want a drug to control them. This desire for a pharmaceutical intervention for teenage angst is another symptom of a major crisis for which the response is clearly inadequate. Owing to the lack of psychiatric beds for hospital care, teenagers deemed by caregivers to be wild and out of control are regularly boarded in emergency departments. In major cities you can find urgent care centers for mental health issues as well as behavioral health urgent care. There are also 24-hour crisis phone lines (988 in the US) to call and mobile teams to come to you. Search the internet for more options! While it can be lifesaving, it is also a limited, individualized way to deal with a collective and systemic problem. That is how we currently address the mental health needs of our society.

The October 16, 2022, *New York Times* entire opinion section was devoted to mental illness. Titled, "It's Not Just You: America's Mental Health Crisis Isn't Just About Feelings. It's About Money, Power and Politics Too," articles looked at politics, culture, race, racism, ethnicity, faith, peak mental health, therapy experiences, recovered memories of repressed early-life events, technological care, suicides, liberal therapists and political conservatives, community mental health, teenagers, and social media. The authors pointed out that the carceral, or prison, system was one of the few places where impoverished people can get mental illness treatment. There are more seriously mentally ill people in American jails and prisons than in hospitals. Why? Recall that people suffering poverty have a higher risk of having a mental illness, and they are also more likely to be in the informal economy, more likely to be criminalized and arrested, and more likely to be shut away in the carceral system (recall that almost 1 in 100 Americans are behind bars). Beginning over 75 years ago, there was a push to empty state hospitals that housed those with mental illness. Today, in our for-profit care system, it is not income-generating to hospitalize immiserated populations. In contrast to the other rich nations, the US has the fewest number of hospital beds of any kind per person, and unlike in the Canadian example cited earlier, this statistic is not associated with lower rates of morbidity or mortality.

In the entire *New York Times* series, there is no mention of how any other country was addressing the problem. American exceptionalism suggests we can't learn from others. The lead article by Danielle Carr, "Mental Health Is Political," pointed out that we live in a society where the social fabric has been destroyed. Our feelings of anxiety and sadness, she suggested, are entirely normal reactions to difficult circumstances and not symptoms of compromised mental health. Medicalizing mental illness doesn't work very well if the goal is to address the underlying cause of our mental and emotional distress. However, for those in power, mental illness treatment in the traditional sense, with drugs and forms of therapy, is a solution that lets ordinary people think something is being done. Just as in *Brave New World* Aldous Huxley presented "soma" as the quick fix, we offer psychoactive drugs to people struggling with psychic and social pain. We must ask serious questions about what is causing our plight and whether long-term solutions require nonmedical or political responses.

The cover story of the May 2023 edition of *The Atlantic* was titled "American Madness." Jonathan Rosen describes the tragic story of his brilliant friend, a schizophrenic, who killed his girlfriend while hallucinating a few decades ago. Now deemed insane, the friend has been locked up in an institution. Rosen points out the inadequate US mental illness care, but nowhere in that article is any mention made of the US having much more mental illness than other nations, as the title might suggest. He mentions New York City trying to support the homeless with serious mental conditions. This in a country that has the most expensive healthcare system in the world, and the most treatment for mental illness, yet fails in the basics of providing food and shelter.

The US Office of the Surgeon General, looking at loneliness and isolation, came out with a 2023 advisory on the healing effects of social connection and community [258]. Recommendations included paid family leave, accessible public transportation, parks, libraries, and reforming digital environments. Its 1999 report on mental illness described how common it was and how important early-life impacts were [259]. There was no mention of prisons as places to get treatment. Typical of federal reports, no comparisons were made with other nations.

The unrecognized pandemic of mental illness in the US is worse than that for COVID-19, for which our outcomes, compared with those of other nations, were disastrous. We have a sick society and must address the social determinants of mental health [260]. Perhaps evolution might help us to understand why our society is driving us crazy.

EVOLUTION AND MENTAL HEALTH

Psychiatrist Dr. Randolph Nesse has presented an evolutionary view of mental illness [261]. He suggests that facilitating fitness during the fetal period and early life enhances our ability to reproduce. Increasing our ability to have progeny later compromises our health, through the chronic diseases of aging. As Charles Darwin showed in his 1859 classic *On the Origins of Species*, we must ensure the survival of our species. What matters most are our reproductive years – and the years leading up to them. Later-life issues – such as mental illnesses that become commoner as we age – may not matter for evolutionary success. Some believe this evolutionary approach can help explain some of the mental ill-health issues in the US.

Depression is very common. Much evidence links income inequality with depression around the world, including across US states. With highly stressful conditions present in society, as expected with today's record inequality, one's mood can be one of sadness and loss of hope, or depression. A depressed person may feel this is not the right time to start a family. Our high prevalence of depression may be one interpretation of America's plummeting fertility, now at a historic low.

Attention deficit hyperactivity disorder has been correlated to maternal stress during a particular period of gestation. Those with the condition are vigilant, have a short attention span, look out for trouble, and react to it.

Anxiety is another common mental health condition that continues to increase. Anxiety is an evolutionary adaptation to enable us to cope with danger. Reacting appropriately to the hazard allows survival [262]. Anxiety is related to stress. Anxiety can be aroused by loud noises, rapidly moving objects, pain, screams, being the object of unsmiling attention among strangers, and being alone in a strange place. These are normal reactions to difficult circumstances, not symptoms of poor mental health. Is the high US level of anxiety and fear healthy?

The mainstream US media focus on news of violence, which creates much fear. Such tactics originated with the Roman Emperor Caligua's maxim, "Let them hate me, so long as they fear me." The credo for news is, "if it bleeds, it leads," and politicians, particularly authoritarian ones, have long recognized the rallying effect of conjuring fear among voters. Enhancing a culture of fear contributes to power for a few, as well as being very profitable, whether in sales of weapons, home protection devices, or pepper sprays. Whether it's fear of crime, fear of difference, or fear of a certain kind of people or belief, we have been intentionally primed to live in fear and seek the comfort of something that will alleviate these fears. These stories of violence or potential violence threatening our safety and "way of life" now play continuously on many media platforms to stoke our fears. Fear in some will lead to anger and to rage. It appears we live in an age of rage.

Such a focus on fear produces much anxiety. There is much to be anxious about while living in the United States. Responses include one of the more commonly prescribed drugs in the US, alprazolam (Xanax®), used to treat anxiety. This will not solve the problem of living in an anxiety- or fear-generating society. A population perspective is necessary to treat anxiety and other mental ills.

TREATING A POPULATION

Health in the United States is mediocre at best. The medical care system is only a small explanatory factor for our disproportionate poor health. The political and economic structure matters most. Similarly, when considering mental health, while the US has the most individual treatment, it also lacks good outcomes. The population itself must be treated.

Mental illness is an increasing problem around the world, so a global political response is required, together with individual care. Traditional community psychiatry is not failing everywhere as it is in the United States. Trieste, a city in Italy, closed its equivalent of US state mental hospitals to concentrate on community integration for those with mental illness. The focus on hospitality rather than hospitalization led to much better rates of recovery [249]. We can consider similar innovations.

What to do for those with mental illness now? How many psychiatric hospital beds is ideal for a population? International surveys suggest the optimum number is 60 per 100,000, and fewer than 15 represents a severe shortage. With increasing closures of facilities for inpatient mental illness care, the American number is in the severe shortage range [249]. Use of prisons and jails is inappropriate [263].

Mental illness is a complex entity. If you or someone you care about has mental illness, I'm not advocating any course of individual treatment. Nor am I doing so for any other health condition in this book. Don't stop whatever treatment you are following unless you have good reason to. Seek out good care, whatever that means to you. My concern here is about broader remedies to the collective social illnesses that ail us and how we can transform our society to live healthier lives. The "medicine" being prescribed in this book is political, and the topic of the next chapter.

CHAPTER EIGHT

The Politics of Being Healthy

All diseases have two causes, one pathological, the other political.

Rudolph Virchow

What people do to be healthy depends on the political circumstances of where they live, including their neighborhood, a square mile around their dwelling, say, their city/county, or the state/province/district. Here I argue that the most important geographic setting is the nation state. If the nation state is not healthy, then none of its components will be as healthy as they could be. Health production begins at the top, or country, and spreads out toward the bottom, or you. Unfortunately, this is not how we are supposed to think in a so-called individualistic society such as the United States.

Suppose what you did as an individual mattered most. There are so many health-conscious people in America that surely one of them must rank among the healthiest people on the planet. While we might debate who is healthier than someone else, there is one incontrovertible fact. The oldest person alive at any one time (one measure of health) is almost never in the US. As I've noted, in most situations richer people have better health than impoverished people. But even rich Americans are not that healthy when compared with people in many other countries.

The political context in which we engage in healthy behaviors matters. By political context, I'm referring to elements of how to govern a society, which includes power and economic relationships.

Most people do not think that one's health primarily depends on political choices. The results of internet surveys that ask Americans to rank 10 determinants of health typically put healthcare first and politics last [32]. When reporting on the 1848 typhus epidemic in Upper Silesia,

Rudolf Virchow, the founder of modern cellular pathology, noted, "Medicine is a social science, and politics nothing but medicine on a grand scale." The term "medicine" as used there means what we call public health today. The statement is often referred to as public health's biggest idea [264]. So just what are the realities of such medicine on a grand scale? Let's begin at the national, or federal, level.

FEDERAL POLITICS AND HEALTH 101

Two themes circulate throughout this book. Inequality in wealth and income is bad for us. And conditions in early life foretell adult health. These two themes are intertwined.

The political structure of a society determines its level of inequality. Consider a state with its citizens. The government commands resources to govern. To govern means to administer or provide services to the inhabitants. Historically, some governments, such as Stalin's USSR, have been very harsh to some of their citizens, but benevolent to others. Recall Tony Benn's description of power. In whose interests is that power exercised, and can the person with power be gotten rid of? If it is not possible to get rid of them, then you do not live in a democracy. The USSR was not a democracy. The United States is assumed to be one. Both autocracies and democracies are different forms of government, yet act in similar ways in many respects. Both types of government can take from the people in the form of taxation and give to the people in the realm of benefits.

International comparisons of key factors help us to understand what is going on. Figure 8.1 illustrates trends in what governments in five nations, Britain, France, Germany, Sweden, and the United States, received in tax revenues from 1870 to 2015 [265]. In the nineteenth century, these governments commanded less than 10% of their nation's economy in taxes. This tax provided a standing army to protect the rulers and paid for their castle (or comparable seat of government). After 1910 they began increasing the government's revenue. By 1980 it rose to a peak, with Sweden receiving close to 55% and the US receiving the least, at 30%. Swedes pay high taxes and receive substantial benefits, such as generous parental leave, free education, housing support, and medical care. They don't complain about paying high taxes as they get much in return. The United States' government collects a much smaller proportion in

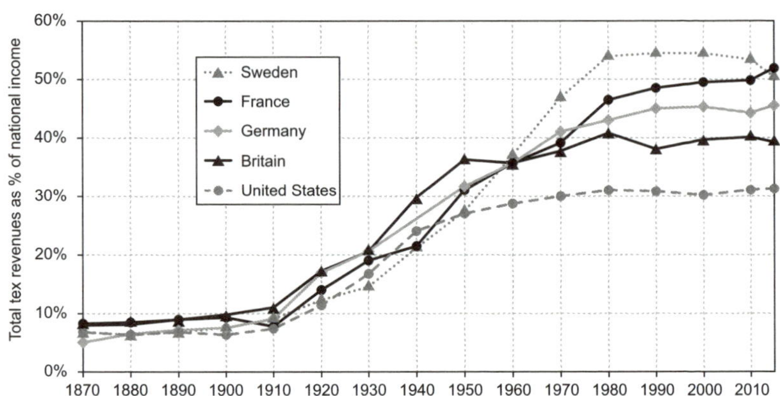

8.1 Rise of the fiscal state in Britain, France, Germany, Sweden, and the United States, 1870–2015 [265]

tax revenue to spend differently. Much goes to the military, close to half of the world's total military expenditures. Another large portion goes to Social Security and Medicare, which mostly benefit people over age 65. Not much goes to the things that improve population health. Given the investment, or lack of investment, our nation makes in our social benefits, let's ask, who pays the bulk of the tax bill these days?

As I've noted, the richest 400 people in the United States pay the lowest tax rate (23% – combined federal, state, and local taxes) of everyone in the country [187]. They receive wealth beyond anyone's dreams, with which they do as they please, yet they contribute the least to the local and federal governments. Back in 1950, the richest 400 paid 70% of their income in taxes. Today the bottom 90% of Americans pay around 28% of their income in taxes. A regressive tax system is where those who earn less (the bottom nine-tenths of Americans) pay more taxes than those with too much (the 400 richest). While this disproportionate wealth certainly gives the rich an advantage, and while there is a health benefit to being rich, why aren't the richest Americans as healthy as less rich Europeans?

Recall our unique failure in providing paid maternity leave to new mothers, which impacts the future health of children who are weaned early and lose that maternal contact. Another factor we might consider is college education, which used to be almost free at a state school and is now exorbitantly expensive. Government expenditures on healthcare per capita are greater than in any other country, yet perhaps a third of Americans have great difficulty accessing needed medical services. This severely affects the bottom 90% of society. The richest do well in these areas as they can afford a parent staying home, college education, and the costs of their medical care, but, as pointed out, they still do not do as well as much less rich folk do in other developed countries.

Defense services provided by the federal government represent almost half of the discretionary budget – nearly a trillion dollars, far more than any other nation spends, and about 40% of the world's total. The other half of discretionary spending are programs for housing and community services, education, healthcare, food assistance, job training and place-ment, unemployment, foreign aid, and scientific research. The huge defense spending represents the interests of the powerful US military–industrial complex. Unlike other discretionary spending, it is not subject to audit.

Consider our own or our family's budget. We estimate what amount of money we will take in from working or from other sources, calculate pro-posed expenditures, where that money will go, and see if something is left over that we can save. We can have a balanced budget, namely earnings equal expenses. Or we might enjoy a surplus, money left over, that leads to savings. If the expenses exceed what we spend, we have a deficit and need another source of money to cover that. Typically, one gets a loan to cover the deficit. That loan may come from a bank, a credit card, or a payday loan company or pawn shop. Payday loans, that is, very short-term loans, are unsecured, meaning you don't have collateral (unlike the pawn shop, where you leave something for the money you receive) for the store to take if you don't pay, so they charge high interest rates over a very short term. There are twice as many such loan sharks than McDonald's restaurants and they are commonly used, especially by younger people and people of color, who are more likely to be paid low wages. One in 20 Americans has taken out a payday loan at some point – 5% of the population – and interest rates can legally go as high as 1,900%! (No, that's not a typo.)

At the federal level, the country does not have to balance its budget. It can spend more than it takes in. It borrows to pay the bills.

This practice leads to the US national debt, which, as of 2024, is over $33 trillion. There is a legislated ceiling to the debt, which Congress must extend regularly as our debt increases. Paying interest on the debt is the third largest federal expenditure of our tax dollars. But back in the 1950s, when the wealthiest paid the most taxes, there was no debt. The debt is higher than our GDP (gross domestic product – the combined value of goods and services in the country). The only other time it was this high was during World War II when we borrowed to pay for that war. Much of the debt goes to pay for our unsuccessful wars in Iraq and Afghanistan (estimated to cost $5 trillion, each), as well as the bailout of the banks in the 2008–9 financial crisis. None of the bankers who were bailed out went to jail; instead, they became richer through our largesse. Debt is debt. Regardless of how we got into debt, there's only one way out of it, and that's paying it.

One way of having less debt is to increase revenue, namely the amount of money brought in to pay for what the government does. For a family budget, if there isn't enough money coming in with one parent working, the other parent goes out and gets a job so together they can pay the bills. Back in 1970, the median (the midpoint, with half above and half below) two-parent, two-child family had one parent working for pay outside the home (usually the father), and the other working at home without receiving a wage (usually the mother).

Senator Elizabeth Warren compared the budget of the 1970 family with a similar 2000 family. In 2000, both parents typically worked outside the home. The 1970 family, with just one parent working outside the home, had enough savings left over to pay for a vacation and other pleasures, unlike the 2000 family with both parents working [266]. Something had changed over those 30 years in American conditions that made it necessary for both parents to work to have enough revenue to pay the bills and not have much left over. Just like the family in 2000, the government could have increased revenue rather than going into greater debt; instead, it chose to decrease revenue mostly by lowering taxes – not on the middle class, but on the wealthiest.

The federal government increases debt mainly by borrowing from countries such as China, rich corporations, and wealthy Americans who invest in government treasuries and bonds. Instead of taxing US entities so that we do not have debt, the government borrows from them and then has to pay them interest on the loan. The annual cost exceeds a trillion dollars. This is a wasteful strategy. It hurts us all, even the wealthy, by increasing inequality, which worsens the health of all of us.

Government revenue comes mostly from various taxes, which include income taxes and payroll taxes, then corporate taxes (quite small today), sales taxes, and customs duties (today called tariffs). Those in power, the rich, prefer to guard their wealth, a proxy for power, and make sure their taxes are not raised. If their taxes were raised, which could eliminate our nation's debt, they couldn't protect all their wealth. But doing so would make this country prosper.

This simple budgetary principle, raising taxes, is almost never discussed regarding the national debt. While most Americans express opinions that the rich should pay more tax, this obvious step is not mentioned. The same is true for so many issues in the United States, such as during the debate regarding the Affordable Care Act, passed in 2010, when single-payer healthcare, which is to say, government-funded healthcare, was "off the table." Other countries face similar situations, but their citizens are not so accepting of fiscal restraint.

Consider France, where the age of retirement has been raised from 62 to 64, when retirees receive a government pension. The government was faced with the choice of taxing the rich more or cutting expenditures on pensions; it did the latter through a nonparliamentary decision, because if it went through the parliament, it would have failed. French citizens protested massively, but ultimately unsuccessfully, marking a shift from that nation's long-standing commitment to a robust social safety net.

Since the 1970s, in the US, we've been making similar decisions, with a massive transfer of wealth from the bottom 90% to the top 1%. Analyses put this wealth pump transfer to be almost $79 trillion [267]. Suppose you laid a stack of freshly minted $100 bills, our largest currency, one on top of another, to represent $79 trillion. It would reach almost 54,000 miles into space – close to a quarter of the way to the moon!

Unlike in France, however, here there is little public protest as we chisel away at our safety net. Here, people are far more likely to protest "spending" – defined as investing in the social safety net and other public goods – than we are to demonstrate for increasing taxes on the richest of the rich. Is this mostly because Americans are unaware of the scale of the heist, or, if they are aware, they don't expect the political system to serve them? Today's political turmoil in the United States suggests it is the latter, though the media, mostly monopolized by a few very wealthy corporations, have distracted us from this pilferage.

Despite this massive transfer of wealth, public opinion polls point out that many Americans consider this wealth transfer to be unfair. Yet in comparisons across nations, according to a recent study where people were shown information about how the economy was rigged to advantage the rich, Americans had much less support for redistribution than people in Australia, France, Germany, Switzerland, or the United Kingdom [268]. Most people here, believing in the American Dream, perceive themselves as upwardly mobile, when, in fact, they are not. Americans see inequality as a gateway to opportunity, requiring personal responsibility, and thus they tolerate these extremes. The study also pointed out how much distrust there is of the US government, which leads to apathy about whether the government should do something about inequality. We have a lose–lose situation.

The second theme, early life, is also not under our individual control. You can't ensure that a couple about to become parents will have had little chronic stress preconception. And during pregnancy, advising parents to just not be stressed won't work. Throughout the rest of the first 1,000 days, you can't make most parents be there for their infants, because they must work to pay the bills or want to pursue careers. So, today's families face budgetary problems that lead to raising children who become less healthy adults than they could be. As with the wealth transfer, most Americans want support for early life in the form of paid parental leave, free or low-cost childcare, and preschool. But such social support, provided in virtually all other rich countries in the world, is said to be too expensive for the US government to provide.

The political system in the United States does not lay the foundation for an early life that leads to healthy adults. Everyone loses. We all lose health, whether we are rich or not so rich. Just as the economy is getting worse, our health, however measured, continues to decline.

What we, the American people, desire – universal healthcare, a social safety net if we lose our homes or jobs, the ability to stay home with our infants and have access to quality, affordable daycare when we return to work – is not what we get, because those wants are off the table for discussion in our political system. But is this political system meeting our needs? Let us explore a comprehensive study done on federal policies and whether they represent the needs of US citizens.

Researchers, Gilens and Page, compared citizens' preferences with those of the economic elites and looked at those of both business and public interest groups. They considered almost 1,800 policy decisions made between 1981 and 2002 for which they had survey data on policy preferences [269]. They found that the policy preferences of the wealthy, or economic elites as they were classified, were mostly adopted. Organized interest groups, especially those representing business, had some impact, while the preferences of average citizens, when they opposed those of the elites, had the least policy impacts:

> ... a proposed policy change with low support among economically-elite Americans (one out of five in favor) is adopted only about 18 percent of the time, while a proposed change with high support (four out of five in favor) is adopted about 45 percent of the time.

Is there a popular democracy in the United States? Powerful actors shape agendas in what policy makers consider. When the majority of citizens disagree with the economic elites, they generally lose, meaning they do not get political policies passed that favor their interests.

The government does not serve most of its citizens. In practically all national elections since its founding, the nonvoters are the biggest demographic. Who doesn't vote in national (or local) US elections? The lower your income, the less likely you are to vote. This economic distinction transcends racial divides. Those households with incomes less than $50,000, which includes almost half of the country, are about half as likely to vote as those making $100,000 or more [270]. Thus, national policies that favor the rich are much more likely to be adopted. With a few notable exceptions, such as Bernie Sanders, most politicians running for office do not talk to or about working-class and unemployed low-income people living in poverty here in the USA. Just as in the media, poverty is much less likely to be the focus.

What about below the national or federal level? US federalism means that whatever policies are not directed by the national government through the constitution become the responsibility of states. Education is omitted from the constitution and thereby becomes a state responsibility. Consequently, this results in tremendous variation among the states in education funding and outcomes. Per-pupil funding varies 2.5-fold between the states. Funds for public education come from local property taxes, which vary enormously between more and less affluent areas, meaning the more expensive your home, the better your schools, and the lower your income, the less money your schools have for teachers, books, science labs, technology, extracurricular activities, and other resources. Other rich countries have a more predistributive form of educational funding to make it more equitable. But our public schools are only one casualty of our national priorities and unique political structure. Let's explore more of the roller coaster of federalism and American politics.

US STATE POLITICS AND HEALTH

We've already noted how national policies mostly favor the interests of the wealthy. But do economic elites have the most say in what policies get enacted at the US state level? There is more leeway in state political outcomes, varying from conservative to liberal orientations. These state-level political decisions impact health dramatically.

Consider US states and their policies affecting health from 1958 to 2017. To make strong comparisons, we use death rates. If you are dead, you can't be healthy. Consider working-age mortality, that is, people aged 25–64, whether men or women, dying of any cause. The increase of deaths in this age range account for much of the overall US health decline, with predominant causes being heart disease, drug overdoses, alcohol, and suicides. In a 2013 survey of Americans' desires for how long they wish to live, the researchers found that 85% wanted to live beyond 78 years. Yet in that year, only 60% of US people achieved that goal [271].

In studies that look at the differences between conservative and liberal states, liberal is defined as expanding state power to regulate and redistribute the economic sector and protect marginalized groups, or restricting state power to punishing deviant social behavior; conservative is defined as the opposite. More liberal state policies regulating firearms, labor, environment, criminal justice, taxes, and tobacco led to a lower mortality rate. If all states had a liberal policy orientation, there would have been over 170,000 fewer working-age deaths in 2019 [271]. If all states had conservative policies that year, more than 215,000 such lives would have been lost. This loss of lives represents a 600 passenger airplane crashing every day, or a tragedy on the scale of 9/11 every five days. Such a catastrophe doesn't make headlines. Instead, it is accepted.

Life expectancy trends, based on state policies, also follow the same pattern [178]. Such liberal policies include paid family and sick leave, minimum wages, disability insurance, assault weapon bans, bans on open gun carry, applying California car emissions standards widely, more progressive income taxes, and repeal of the death penalty. Unsurprisingly, our longest-lived state, Hawai'i, has liberal political policies. So why can't we enact laws and policies to address these issues at the federal level?

Governments are designed to move slowly. The US federal government has two branches in Congress: the House of Representatives and the Senate. Legislation must be approved by both branches to become law. That is a slow process that can take years, and often goes nowhere whenever one political party loses control over the House or Senate and another party gains control, quashing the political goals of the previous party.

The only time governments move quickly is when there is some major shock and there is a policy draft ready to spring onto the public. An example is the Patriot Act of 2001 that was ushered in quickly after New York's World Trade Center towers were hit. Such legislation, to counter terrorism in the US and around the world, had been proposed long before, in the hope that an opportunity would come along to enact it. It was passed quickly and the US invaded Afghanistan that year, and then Iraq in 2003. Barring such exceptional circumstances, governmental change is slow.

Blending federal policies with those at the state level provides overwhelming support for politics as the most important determinant of health. Creating this awareness among people in the United States and elsewhere is the critical challenge. Americans tend to think healthcare is what we need for good health, and they consistently rank politics at the bottom of that list [32]. But as I've shown, political issues are the most important determinant of health. How did we get to have policies so detrimental to our health?

MEDICAL CARE VERSUS PUBLIC HEALTH SPENDING

American public health investments (preventive care considered broadly as a public good) lack a constituency to support them, resulting in fewer incentives to pay for such outlays despite substantial benefits. Preventive care covers the broader spectrum of what can be done to make the population healthy besides providing medical or curative care. By contrast, curative care is typically paid for either out of pocket, or by public or mandatory private insurance.

Compared with other rich nations, the United States spends little on preventive or public health expenditures, in contrast to what is spent on healthcare. Spending on curative care has short-term perceived personal benefits for those who see themselves as sick, whereas preventive care benefits unfold in the long term to everyone. The strong advocacy or public interest group support for curative care is lacking for public health. Despite austerity and government spending cuts, people still pay for the perceived benefits of curative healthcare.

Medical care policies are "loud policies" – they appear to offer benefits that mobilize voters, lobby groups, and political parties [272]. Curative healthcare is loud and salient in the public discourse since healthcare needs cover a risk shared by all citizens. Most citizens, regardless of their income or ideology, favor additional spending for curative healthcare. Some loud policies are more divisive, such as unemployment insurance, which offers short-term benefits to a subset of the population and is more likely to be supported by progressive voters and parties on the left, than by the conservative on the right, since it protects people more vulnerable to the risk of job loss.

What should be done to improve US healthcare? We can begin by redesigning the medical education system to make primary care, the most valuable part of healthcare, the principal means of service provision [40,41]. For example, we could provide free medical school tuition for those who agree to provide primary care services after they complete training in a national healthcare services corp. We could decentralize healthcare worker education so training takes place where the need for services exists. The US government already spends more on healthcare per person than any nation that has universal healthcare, so we can afford a single-payer system without additional costs. A healthcare information system is needed that services the patient, family, and interprofessional care team, rather than the billing industry. Even with such a comprehensive transformation, however, population health improvements will be modest at best. Unfortunately, such changes will be strongly resisted, given the pressures and inducements the insurance and healthcare industries exert on lawmakers to maintain the current system.

Then there are "quiet policies" that produce good population health outcomes. Quiet policies support early life, families, those with disabilities, and those who are unemployed by providing sickness cash benefits, employment programs, housing support, and other such assistance. In the public's mind, such policies confuse people and are considered to provide unclear benefits. Even though these policies require relatively low expenditures, they are characterized as "entitlements" that constitute government waste and high spending. They also receive less media attention. Quiet policy advocacy and interest groups, though they may be vocal, do not engage the public as much as the powerful professional lobbyists and organizations do.

Many Americans are not aware of the incredible influence wielded by professional lobbying groups in the US. Those active at the federal level in Washington, DC, must register and file reports of who they represent. This is a requirement for most US states as well, but activity disclosure varies. In Washington state where I live, the names and contact numbers of lobbyists, their firms, and their clients are available on the internet.

The number of federal lobbyists registered with the US Congress keeps rising every year and is close to 13,000, or about 25 per member of the House or Senate. Centered in about 300 lobbying firms that spend over $4 billion, corporate lobbying represents a significant persuasive force in the country, in addition to those at the state, county, and local levels.

International students who come to study at our global health department typically describe corruption in their home country as the biggest problem. When asked what corruption looks like there, what they describe mirrors lobbying in the United States. I tell them the only difference here is that lobbying is legal [273]. They find this difficult to believe.

Major lobby efforts are centered around drugs, pharmaceuticals, and medical products; healthcare guilds, hospitals, and insurance companies; the big internet giants; and real estate agents. Recent investigative reporting has disclosed that elected members of Congress have served on the board of the National Rifle Association (NRA) and actively promoted the unrestricted availability and use of firearms. There is no honor system in place in American politics.

The COVID-19 pandemic brought loud issues to the forefront with high rates of hospitalizations, patients on ventilators, and early deaths. Physical distancing, masking, and vaccinations, public health (or quiet) issues, were deemed unimportant by many Americans who felt these preventive measures were ineffective and/or conflicted with their perceived personal freedoms.

This dismissive stance toward public health is reflected in the scientific process itself. Research on health at the federal level by the National Institutes of Health (NIH) promotes individual health rather than studying communities or states. The proportion of NIH-funded projects with "public" or "population" in the title dropped 90% during the 10 years ending in 2015. The research focus is instead on personalized treatment, especially looking at impacting genomic diseases to decrease health inequities [274]. As important as such treatment may be, ultimately, as long as the individual remains the focus of healthcare, we will not attain health in the country.

Consider the ratio of spending on social expenditures to spending on healthcare among the countries in the Organisation for Economic Co-operation and Development (OECD). This forum compiles data on rich countries. Elizabeth Bradley and her colleagues at Yale looked at the ratio of such quiet policy outlays to outlays on loud policies on curative care. The other healthier nations spent much more on social expenditures than on medical care, while it was the opposite for the US [275]. Whether we call them social or public health or preventive expenditures, this chasm between loud and quiet policies answers the paradox of why we spend so much on healthcare and get so little health.

The question is, why are Americans so reluctant to accept these policies that have such a great and beneficial impact on our health? The answer lies in understanding how our political ideology has changed over the last century.

TRENDS IN THE US POLITICAL LANDSCAPE

Economic and political systems began with the hunter-gatherer era, our longest and most successful form of societal organization characterized by ubiquitous sharing. The dawn of agriculture brought exploitation, with attendant power relationships that led to hierarchy and inequality. Feudalism in various forms dominated the world for centuries.

Feudalism gave way to capitalism with the industrial revolution in Europe. Since its founding, the United States has followed principles of capitalism with various forms, one of which used enslaved workers. While stirrings of socialism began to permeate the country, private enterprise with generous government subsidies became entrenched. Capitalism, as a world system, is a form of labor exploitation and surplus extraction with a focus on profits that predominates today.

Yet capitalism may be nearing the end of its lifespan. The current unstable human situation on the planet with its political turmoil, wars, vastly increasing economic inequality, climate catastrophe, and even declining health are evidence of this. Yanis Varoufakis argues that a system he calls technofeudalism is replacing it [276]. Forms of socialism also contend for how human society may reorganize itself. Capitalism's days are numbered.

After the 1929 stock market crash and the ensuing Great Depression, there came a period of rising labor power with a desire to avoid the economic inequality of the roaring twenties that led to that debacle. President Franklin Delano Roosevelt (FDR) wanted to save capitalism at any cost. He enacted New Deal policies such as federal works programs employing over 10 million people, strengthening the power of labor unions, passing social security legislation to provide pensions for the elderly, as well as unemployment and disability insurance, and enacting legislation to stabilize the economy. To pay for these initiatives he raised taxes on the rich and pointed out to them that this would avoid a revolution. The highest marginal tax rate is what the richest pay on income above a certain amount. Roosevelt wanted that rate to be 100% on incomes over $25,000, effectively making $25,000 a maximum wage (equivalent to over $450,000 today) [277]. While that legislation didn't pass, a law enacted in 1944 put the highest marginal tax rate at 94%. It was raised to 96% in 1946 and remained over 90% in the 1950s. People in the poorest fifth of the United States saw the greatest income gains during that period.

The rich, even though they had much more than before, were unsurprisingly not happy with this situation. They began scheming to lower their federal tax burden. By the 1960s, they'd achieved a drop in the highest marginal tax rate to 70%. The highest federal marginal tax rate was eventually brought down even further to below 40% today. Don't confuse this with the lower rate of combined federal, state, and local taxes for the richest 400 families [187]. This assault on our tax base has produced stratospheric increases in economic inequality, yet few Americans today are even aware that the wealthiest once paid so much more in taxes than they do today.

Major political trends since World War II included a focus on government spending for the common good that began with FDR. Economist John Maynard Keynes considered such spending to increase demand and lead to high employment rates. Milton Friedman and the Chicago School of Economics attacked Keynesian ideas as a failure, which led to the birth of our neoliberal era.

Neoliberalism takes the prefix neo- (meaning new) along with liberalism, to mean readopting nineteenth-century free-market capitalism, characterized by deregulation, privatization, and reductions in government spending. Remove market regulations, they reason, and get the government out of people's lives to let the so-called free market work its miracles. Tracing the wealth of the richest 1% of Americans from the 1920s to the present demonstrates these changes. In the 1920s, the richest 1% had close to half of all wealth, but by 1975 their share had dropped to less than 25% owing to the various redistributive policies propagated by FDR and subsequent leaders [278]. With the neoliberal economics assault, the richest 1% have regained their wealth share. The resulting inequality is one reason why our health in the United States has declined.

Another political realignment took place in the United States in the 1960s, involving both the Democrat and Republican parties, that strongly affected health. The Democratic Party abandoned its support for discriminating against Black peoples. After the Democratic Party embraced the civil rights movement, many Whites moved to the Republican Party, which became increasingly focused on the rights of Whites, limiting affirmative action, controlling women's rights to their reproduction, and promoting lowering taxes on the wealthiest in the name of controlling Democrat spending. The Democrats, meanwhile, promoted neoliberal policies such as the North American Free Trade Agreement (NAFTA), which contributed to the collapse of the manufacturing sector, while also enacting "welfare reform" that limited the safety net for the poorest. Now its ideology is closer to that of the Republican Party, which has become even more socioeconomically and racially conservative. What does this shift in political parties tell us about health? Let's consider infant mortality.

Infant mortality rates (IMRs) are a very sensitive health indicator. From the 1920s, Republican state and national administrations had smaller improvements in infant deaths than Democratic ones, and greater racial gaps [279]. Beginning in the 1970s, however, with the Republicans advocating for more conservative racial policies, Black and White IMRs began to diverge, worsening among Black infants. Infant deaths among Black people in both the Southern States (Confederacy) and non-southern states stopped declining after 2010. There were improvements in this period for White people in the non-southern states, but not for White people in the more racially conservative Southern States. Uniformly, Black people continue to have higher rates of infant deaths than White peoples. For 2022, the Black IMR was twice that of Whites. The difference represents over seven Black infants dying every day who wouldn't die if they had the White IMR. This discrepancy epitomizes structural racism. Just as with adult mortality across states, political policies, laws, and practices reflecting partisan politics strongly impact our infants' health.

Neoliberal economics formally took hold in the late 1970s, but the transformative movement, with the rich wanting ever more, had been there since the end of World War II. A 1948 US State Department Planning Study was explicit [280]:

> [The US has] about 50% of the world's wealth but only 6.3% of its population. . . . In this situation, we cannot fail to be the object of envy and resentment. Our real task in the coming period is to devise a pattern of relationships which will permit us to maintain this position of disparity without positive detriment to our national security.

America's national and foreign policies have been about maintaining US wealth concentration globally. The challenge was to bring the American public on board to let the rich have everything. A *Business Week* story published in 1974 warns of the future [281]:

> It will be a hard pill for many Americans to swallow – the idea of doing with less so that big business can have more . . . Nothing that this nation, or any other nation, has done in modern economic history compares in difficulty with the selling job that must be done to make people accept the new

reality. ... Historian Arnold Toynbee ... laments that democracy will be unable to cope with approaching economic problems – and that totalitarianism will take its place.

Alex Carey, an Australian sociologist, said the twentieth century will be remembered for three major developments. The first was democracy, the second was the rise of huge corporations with their power, and the third was the use of corporate propaganda, public relations, to protect corporate power from democracy [282].

Over the last 60 years we've seen a rightward shift in politics. President Eisenhower, a Republican, was president in the 1950s. Today, he would be considered a liberal, comparable to Bernie Sanders or Alexandria Ocasio-Cortez. He expanded social security, resisted tax cuts, and warned of a growing military–industrial complex. Many policies supported by Republican President Nixon from 1969 to 1974, such as environmental protection laws, occupational safety legislations, and policies pertaining to welfare, traffic safety, and equal rights, would be considered left wing today.

An assault on democracy followed the 1975 publication of the Trilateral Commission's report [283]. It suggested there could be too much people power, as was evident in the 1960s, leading to "an excess of democracy" and called for a "greater degree of moderation" in democracy.

President Reagan accelerated the attack on democracy. He advocated "trickle-down" economics by drastically cutting taxes on rich people, ostensibly so they would invest more of their wealth to produce more jobs for the rest of us. Reagan used racism as a political wedge to erode White majority support for Aid to Families with Dependent Children (AFDC) – the primary government program providing cash assistance to poor families with children. He deployed the Black "welfare queen" stereotype, implying that everyone on welfare was Black and drove around in Cadillacs exploiting the system, and suggesting that public assistance and, at the same time, Black, impoverished people and communities were a moral hazard. If we help "the poor," whom his racist rhetoric about welfare conveniently coded as Black, Reagan reasoned, they won't have any incentive to work. The selling job to the US public was highly successful, and people paradoxically supported lower taxes on the rich while their share of the tax bill increased.

This rightward geopolitical shift continued with President George HW Bush, then Presidents Bill Clinton and George W Bush. Clinton's policies of welfare reform ("the end of welfare as we know it"), ending the Glass–Steagall Act that separated investment and commercial banking, and the "three strikes and you're out" prison reform that sent people to prison for life for minor crimes led to both economic crises and poverty increases that devastated communities. Although President Obama promised "hope and change," neoliberal economics remained his agenda. President Trump further intensified these trends. He also set back much past progress. The COVID-19 outcomes in the United States were among the worst in the world, both in infection rates and in deaths. Moreover, his attack on vaccines as an attack on "freedom" has led to calls to end all vaccine mandates in public schools. We are consequently seeing a surge in measles across the nation, as parents refuse to vaccinate children against this deadly, but almost eradicated, contagious disease. Public health policies, always quiet, have been retrenched, making us more vulnerable to the next contagion. After all these "reforms," we have more poverty than any other rich nation.

Many Americans struggle daily just to pay the rent. How will they pay the heating bill, or the light bill, or buy groceries to feed their children? We must understand their plight. Yet too often, politicians weaponize poverty against their political foes, not presenting effective policies to address it, but blaming the other party for poverty's existence or its social impacts. Politics is broken in America. Consider January 6, 2021.

The storming of the US Capitol on January 6, 2021, to overturn the election resulted from the lie being spread from the highest offices that the 2020 election was stolen. Despite every court and audit challenge finding no merit to the claim, a large proportion of Americans, and especially Republicans, still believe this lie. With Trump's "Make America Great Again" (MAGA) slogan, he has effectively organized blue-collar White men as his base. Between 2008 and 2018, median incomes in Democratic congressional districts rose from $54,000 to $61,000, while in Republican districts they fell from $55,000 to $53,000. Health is worse in Republican districts. Rural White Americans report less optimism about the future as well [284]. Trump moved the conversation from losing to stealing, presenting Heroic America, White power, old-time manhood, and other attributes as all stolen from the country.

RACISM AND GENDER INEQUITIES

Today in the US we face culture war issues among political tribes, some of whom fuel neofascist ideology; others propel nationalism, xenophobia, anti-immigration, racial supremacy, and authoritarianism. Cooperation with other nations has dwindled. We live in a precarious state. Consider racism in America today.

Borrowing from Dr. Camara Jones, we can describe racism as a gardener's tale [285]. A gardener plants seeds from two different packages, one for red flowers and one for pink flowers, in two different potting soils. The soil where the red flower seeds go has been newly purchased. The other pot contains last year's soil. The red flowers produce abundantly, while the pink flowers do not do as well. Forgetting the soil differences, she concludes that red flowers are superior to pink ones and focuses her care and attention on the red flowers. If a pink flower seed is blown into the better soil, the gardener plucks the flower out before it can establish itself.

Personally mediated colorism is picking out the less attractive colored flower. By contrast, structural or institutional racism is not recognizing the soil differences that produced the two different colored flowers. The soils of racism have been unequal since enslavement. Due to racism and its explicit goal of maintaining the exploitability of certain communities' labor and laborers, Black unemployment always remains higher than that of other groups, and Black people's incomes have mostly stagnated, while those of White people have risen [286]. Black people's median net wealth has remained just above zero (meaning debts and assets cancel each other) while White median net wealth has more than doubled to over $150,000 since the 1980s [286]. Perpetuating concepts of innate racial differences leads to the devastating impact of ongoing racialized social, physical, and institutional violence, and the economic violence of deep income and wealth inequality on our health.

One response to the enslavement of Black Americans is to consider reparations for the sins of our forefathers [287,288].The California legislature is considering payments, such as tuition or housing grants, and even direct cash payments, to descendants of enslaved African Americans. William Darity Jr. of Duke University proposes taking excess White wealth in the US today and transferring it so African Americans who had one enslaved ancestor receive enough to eradicate the racial wealth gap [289]. Many Democrats and Black Americans favor reparations, less so Republicans and White people who enjoy their privileges and are hesitant to lose any.

Consider gender disparities. What about women who have gained rights and participate in politics?

Data from 49 European countries show that greater political participation by women leads to better health for everyone [290]. Measured by the percentage of national parliamentary seats held by women, the benefits of greater representation of women include better health for both men and women and smaller health inequalities between men and women. The gender equality benefits include less harm from air pollution and smaller geographical differences in IMRs. Worldwide, only a handful of countries have half of parliamentary seats held by women. Greater female political participation is good for everyone's health.

American women's political status is behind that of so many other nations. Women make up about a quarter of the US Congress. Kamala Harris was the first woman vice president. Unlike so many other nations, the United States has never had a woman president. Women still earn about three-quarters of a man's salary, and this proportion is even smaller for women of color. Appalachia and the southeastern states, with the most conservative political policies, have the least female power and the worst health.

OPEN-AND-SHUT CASE AGAINST INEQUALITY

With so much evidence about the harms of racialized and gendered economic inequality, there should be no doubt about reducing that bane [291]. Discussions and debate must move beyond economics for a multidisciplinary approach of the impacts on health to persuade the public. The public must understand how economic inequality is bad for everyone. But drawing attention to economic issues is difficult.

Relative deprivation is a research term used to gauge inequality. In the absence of absolute deprivation, meaning incomes are inadequate to meet an adequate standard of living, upward income comparisons damage health, well-being, and life satisfaction. A big income gap does not produce human flourishing, because people make upward comparisons, namely no matter how much they have, it is never enough, in comparison to keeping up with the Jones'.

As I've shown, decreasing inequality will produce healthy changes in the United States. So how do we accomplish this?

CHAPTER NINE

Ineffective Health Production Efforts

If you keep on doing what you've always done, you will keep getting what you've always gotten.

Henry Ford

The health calamity in the United States has been going on for more than 50 years. What began as a relative decline, namely our health was not improving as much as that of many other nations, has for the past decade become an absolute decline, that is, death rates are going up. During this period there have been many efforts that supposedly were to improve our health and well-being but have clearly not worked. Studying those will steer us toward other measures that will work.

Producing health is a political process, as outlined in the previous chapter. The policies in place, namely those that transfer wealth to the richest, and serve the rich, aren't effective health policies. Similarly health policies that beneficially impact early life are absent here.

Spending huge amounts on medical care likewise distracts us from effective ways to improve health.

Those who influence the political process, lobbyists, mostly retard health, but further neoliberalism, which enhances the profits of large corporations that wield the most power. Public health policies, quiet in nature, need to be emboldened by population health strategies.

To change policy, we have to understand the process of producing policy.

POLICY STEPS

Gilens and Page discovered that elites get the policies that benefit them in the short run, making it difficult to get the policy changes that are required to improve US health [269]. Despite their advantages, the health of our nation's elites is compromised just by being here. They don't know this morbid fact. They want to live longer, healthier lives. They need to be convinced of the risks they face by living here. Then there will be hope for policies to improve *their* health! But how to convince them that living in the US worsens their health? This is described in the next chapter.

Few readers of this book will be among those economic elites. Reaching them requires growing a national movement like that to deal with our climate crisis. What ignites action, however, tends to be violent and visible, such as the 2020 police murder of George Floyd. Our declining health is not predominantly such visible violence, but structural violence and social murder, as described below.

We are dying from the usual causes such as heart disease, cancer, and other chronic conditions. Impoverishment is a leading cause of death [292], but it is hard to get people to focus on this fact. To those who do not see themselves as poor, they think that reason doesn't apply to them. This is a mistaken idea, since the underlying mechanisms producing health inequalities and disparities are grotesque economic inequality and lack of attention to early life, which worsens everyone's health. Yet these quiet ideas do not garner attention.

The pace leading to illness and disease is slow and different from an obvious killing. There is no bullet hole nor smoking gun. Social murder was the term applied by Friedrich Engels when discussing English workers, as he wrote in *The Condition of the Working Class in England in 1844* [293]:

When society places hundreds of proletarians in such a position that they inevitably meet a too early and an unnatural death, one which is quite as much a death by violence as that by the sword or bullet; when it deprives thousands of the necessaries of life, places them under conditions in which they cannot live – forces them, through the strong arm of the law, to remain in such conditions until that death ensues which is the inevitable consequence – knows that these thousands of victims must perish, and yet permits these conditions to remain, its deed is murder ... society in England daily and hourly commits what the working-men's organs, with perfect correctness, characterise as social murder ... it has placed the workers under conditions in which they can neither retain health nor live long.

In trying to understand such violence, I came across the phrase structural violence, in contrast to behavioral or physical violence. The behavioral version is obvious, typically from a personal act by a perpetrator that injures someone or damages something. Structural violence causes injury or damage not from the act or acts of individuals, but from political and social structures of institutions and other frameworks of society, leading to various forms of inequality. It is invisible, being built into the fabric of society and thus escapes recognition. There is no smoking gun. It is like social murder [294]. This insidious concept, comparable to social murder, resides in a quiet space hidden from our consciousness.

MAJOR PARADIGM SHIFTS

What produces major changes in how people think and see the world? Consider attempts made to keep secret the explosion of the first atomic bomb in New Mexico on July 16, 1945. Only after a bomb was dropped on Hiroshima on August 6, 1945, were events made public. *The New York Times* for August 7, 1945, had the headline, "First Atomic Bomb Dropped on Japan; Missile Is Equal to 20,000 Tons of TNT; Truman Warns Foe of a 'Rain of Ruin'." The article then mentioned for the first time that there had been a previous test. Our War Department (today renamed the Department of Defense) called it a cosmic bomb. The bombing was done after America received word that Japan was willing to surrender on the condition that their emperor not be executed. However, we wanted to show the world our new lethal device. Pictures of the mushroom cloud soon followed. Our world had entered a new era through a new technology, one that God should not have given. This is an example of behavioral violence. The damage was visible, rapid, and devastating.

Other examples of visible behavioral violence, such as the coffins of US soldiers returning from Vietnam, led to changes in journalism during the American invasions of Afghanistan and Iraq. Then, in Afghanistan and Iraq, embedded journalists were the only conduits for news, which was carefully sanitized to not show our troop casualties. This contrasts heavily with the Russian invasion of Ukraine and the situation in Gaza and Israel, where gruesome headlines are seen daily. The news we are exposed to has become increasingly crafted to serve imperial hegemonic interests.

Metaphors of structural violence, such as the US carnage being equivalent to the 2001 World Trade Center towers collapsing every five days, do not catch attention. In the previous chapter we talked about avoidable deaths in the US being equivalent to a 600 passenger airplane crashing every day. This is what the arithmetic shows, but it does not move the heart into action.

How we can persuade ordinary people, and the economic elites, to recognize that they are affected by structural violence, or social murder, is the subject of the next chapter. Even the elites must come to see that their greed is killing them through many channels. And we must get our leaders on board. But there are major forces at work to distract us from social murder, including charities and philanthropies.

PHILANTHROPY AND CHARITY

The charity industry, a legacy of colonialism, represents the paternalistic mindset of helping. Philanthropy is an expression of elite power over the public, typically depending on the personal whims of the superrich. The US has about 10 times more such beneficence than other rich nations. But there is no such thing as a free gift. Where do these discretionary contributions go? They disproportionately go to those with much money: private foundations, then colleges and universities, then hospitals and medical centers. In 2019, orphanages got less than a 60th of donations to foundations [295]. In 2022 an estimated 41% of individual donations going to charity went to either a private foundation or a donor-advised fund (DAF) [296].

Donor-advised funds are the most rapidly growing recipient of charity funds, now representing a quarter of all donations. They have considerable tax benefits and secrecy protections, and are not required to pay out any amount. Their sponsors (Fidelity, Schwab, Vanguard) take in more money than the largest public charities. There are no data on payout rates as they are not required to report them. One report showed over a third did not pay out any money to charity in a given year, and in California from 2016 to 2020, almost half of DAFs paid out less than 5% in any given year.

Foundations are required to annually pay out a certain small proportion (no less than 5%) of their endowment. The largest foundations stick closely to that limit, which can include contributing to DAFs. The return on their investment is typically greater than what they disburse, so despite their distributions, they get bigger and more powerful over time. The payout includes their administrative expenses (which can include massive lobbying campaigns), rents, and salaries, as well as support for trustees, which don't directly benefit recipients.

There are well over 100,000 private foundations in America. Foundations mostly advance conservative causes that elites favor. The American Enterprise Institute and the Heritage Foundation push for neoliberal causes. So-called liberal philanthropies that purport to help the poor in the developing world typically do so by promoting shifts from subsistence multicrop agriculture, which sustains rural communities, to export monocrop agriculture, which requires wage labor, chemical inputs, irrigation, and other costly items that demands purchasing Western goods. At the domestic level, high salaries paid to educated professionals tend to be prioritized over the money that reaches the poorest members of society. And many liberal foundations provide direct services rather than advocate for policy changes.

Philanthropies are largely unaccountable to the public, and accountable just to their trustees. Rob Reich points out that philanthropies are not transparent, with many not even having a website [297]. Philanthropy undermines equality. They are heavily subsidized by the public, costing the US Treasury more than $100 billion annually in lost tax revenue. Yet there is virtually no call to make philanthropies more accountable to the public, nor to address the underlying political forces that drive the need for philanthropy in the first place, such as addressing why people are hungry or without homes [298]. We even hear more calls by those on the conservative right to cut the social safety net our government provides and expand philanthropy!

Nor can we depend on churches and volunteers to take up the slack to make America healthy again. Piecemeal voluntary efforts by compassionate conservatives, that is, those who favor limited government support for the disadvantaged, cannot make up for what governments fail to do, namely addressing poverty, declining health, and homelessness, and providing early-life benefits and other supports that other rich countries provide.

Socially responsible investing (SRI) and impact investing, striving for positive social impacts, are vanity concepts. Businesses said to be socially responsible strive for substantial profits. No inroads resulted after the banking crisis in 2008 nor the more recent absolute US health decline. In our capitalist system, social investing is a myth.

Gift-giving and fundraising are now taught in universities, yet all too often these departments are closely tied to the corporate world, where corporations define the priorities and values that underlie philanthropy. Indiana University hosts the Lilly Family School of Philanthropy offering undergraduate degrees up to a doctorate in philanthropy. Lilly is the incredibly profitable drugmaker that made modern, synthesized insulin unaffordable. President Biden's 2023 State of the Union address called for lowering the price of insulin. Lilly, in response and from pressure by US state governments, subsequently lowered the price for those with healthcare insurance, but not for others. Its profits continue to rise. Across the nation, philanthropy and fundraising are becoming popular professions that attract liberal scholars, while shaping them to be corporate professionals. There is a questionable benefit.

Consider nonprofit or 501(c)(3) tax-exempt organizations in the United States. They are not taxed. To keep their nontaxable status, these organizations cannot be overtly political. Such do-gooders are some of our largest employers. The bulk of nonprofits are in the northeast, and the region with the smallest proportion is the southeast, where the need is greatest. I'm not implying that these entities do not do good, but their efforts are not going to regain the lost health in America. (I belong to one such organization, Washington Physicians for Social Responsibility, so I'm not immune to being involved.)

With so many charitable organizations trying to do good in America, recent events, such as the banking crisis in 2008 when the government bailed out the bankers rather than those whose homes were foreclosed, and the debacle over the COVID-19 pandemic when over 1.1 million deaths occurred in the US – the most of any country – suggest our system of relying on nonprofits is not working. Our system is the sickness. In his 1981 inaugural address, President Ronald Reagan said, "Government is not the solution to our problem, government *is* the problem." That statement launched the antigovernment conservative (used in the same sense as above) tide that has demonized any effort by the government to provide for its citizens, from chipping away at our environmental protections, workplace safety, and the social safety net, to current efforts to undermine any corporate oversight. Government efforts now mostly increase the wealth of the richest and foster a system that leads to us being born sick.

If the charitable contributions went into the government revenue stream as taxes and other transfers instead of foundations, the public could democratically decide how the money is spent, so more might go to lessen poverty and inequality.

A few ultrarich have coined the term "giving pledge" to lessen their wealth remorse. These billionaires give on the order of 0.1% of their wealth in any given year. The 73 giving pledgers in 2010 saw their wealth grow by 224%, adjusted for inflation through 2022. Most give to their own private foundations. Some of the wealthiest people who have made this pledge live in Washington state where they do not have to pay a state income tax on the income they derive from their wealth. Consider this charitable–industrial complex their guilt-washing station or reputation launderer that further enhances their wealth. A 6% annual wealth tax would raise 100 times more.

As an example, Jeff Bezos' wealth is about $220 billion. A 6% wealth tax would generate $13 billion annually. This tax would have no impact on his lifestyle and little effect of a small decline in wealth. He could continue spending billions of dollars on luxury real estate and other baubles, as well as his space venture. His wealth would increase substantially through payments of cloud rent, the technofeudalism concept presented above and detailed below [276], which is how Amazon gets richer.

With an additional $13 billion accruing annually to the federal government, this could pay for over 30,000 home units (assuming an average cost of $250,000 per unit) to make a dent in America's huge housing insecurity.

This is just applying the tax on one person. America's billionaires have a combined wealth of over $6 trillion. Taxing this at 6% would provide $360 billion annually that the federal government could use to end homelessness, decrease or eliminate poverty, or fund a national paid parental leave program, among many choices that could be made democratically.

Philanthropies allow their donors not only to avoid taxation of their wealth, but also to decide how their wealth is used. The Gates Foundation represents vanity charity. Messianic Bill Gates is not accountable to anyone except the court of public opinion, while public relations professionals glorify him worldwide. Tim Schwab looks at these myriad aspects [299]. The foundation's self-generated publicity points to saving millions and millions of lives. Gates takes credit for having saved the lives of 122 million children in the past 25 years. He comes to this number by looking at what the child mortality rates used to be and what they are now. Schwab speaks to the ability of the world's most powerful private foundation to shape what we know and how we think. The Gates-funded Institute for Health Metrics and Evaluation (IHME) at the University of Washington is a source for many data presented in my book. One of the world's leading medical journals, *The Lancet*, publishes much of the IHME's results. Its so-called peer-reviewed articles – a questionable process since much of the material in a paper resides in hundreds of pages of accompanying notes – are unlikely to be scrupulously reviewed.

Living in Seattle I find it difficult to get folks here or anywhere to look above the halo over Gates' head, as people assume he is doing so much good. Many are reluctant to criticize Bill Gates or his foundation, self-censorship termed the Bill Chill, as they don't want to bite the hand that feeds them. The foundation has donated billions to universities. At the University of Washington, there are several buildings funded by Gates or the Gates Foundation, displaying their family names. Along with other institutes and entities here, I essentially work at Gates University.

The power and influence of the Gates Foundation is greater than that of the World Health Organization, and likely also the United Nations and major governments, perhaps even the United States. This should make us very uncomfortable. Where its money goes is not transparent. Recall Tony Benn's questions about power presented in Chapter 5: Where do you get it? In whose interests do you exercise it? To whom are you accountable? And how can we get rid of you [179]? The foundation's power resides in its wealth, which is not accountable to we, the people, nor to anyone. There is no mechanism to get rid of it.

Gates voices strong feelings about protecting intellectual property rights and looking for technological solutions to problems. He is the same person who cofounded Microsoft and led it to become a corporate monopoly. There he bullied and lambasted others who had finite greed. Today he remains a corporate opportunist. He funds the rich, mostly wealthy, White-dominated institutions (residing largely in the US and Europe) to help address overseas impoverished communities and populations. None of the foundation's board of directors resides in poor nations. That model of America's rich trying to help those less fortunate doesn't work in the United States. What would be different in poor countries?

In 2022, the cost to the people for supporting the ultra-wealthy philanthropists was over $110 billion in tax revenue loss that we could have potentially controlled. This is without including capital gains revenue lost from the donation of appreciated assets. Philanthropies are a policy-obstruction network. We could use these funds for social spending that does make a difference. We need higher taxes on the rich.

To move beyond the nonprofit and charity–industrial complex, we must work together, since we, the people, have theoretical power that we don't recognize. Our individual rights and freedoms do not add up to collective power. Working together we can gain political power, and we can accomplish the transition to a healthy society [300]. That requires solidarity rather than charity. Once we recognize that the power of the people is greater than the power of the people in power, together we can take on the power brokers and be freed.

Charity is a paradox: the Brazilian Catholic Archbishop Dom Hélder Câmara said, "When I give food to the poor, they call me a saint. When I ask why the poor have no food, they call me a communist."

Charity and philanthropy are essential to the maintenance and perpetuation of the economic elites and the economic and social policies that benefit and enrich them. We need to go beyond such organizations that don't address key health issues in the US. Consider what belongs or should belong to the people.

WHOM SHOULD US RESOURCES BENEFIT?

The land that comprises the United States was taken from the indigenous inhabitants beginning with the arrival of British settlers by 1585, with the first permanent settlement said to have been started in 1607. There followed centuries of genocide through direct violence, bioterrorism (exposure to lethal diseases), and other forms of extermination. The United States was founded in 1776. In recent years, various meetings may begin with a performance of the land acknowledgment ritual. Namely the event is taking place on stolen land, although the language may be softened considerably. It implies that the natives have disappeared, which is far from the truth. Although vastly reduced in numbers, American Indians, as they are called, remain and have the worst health outcomes in the USA. The history of enslavement produced immense wealth. Today those residing in America can claim immense resources.

If today we own something valuable that generates income or profits, who is entitled to that gain? If the answer is, "we are," then what happens when that "we" is a nation? Who should benefit from what belongs to the people? Many productive resources reside in the United States. The oil in the soil, the transcendent power of the airwaves, and the wealth of the national forests are ours. Oil is a vital resource laid down millions of years ago; much progress has been made exploiting this cheap, but exhaustible, resource. In Texas, this resource is considered to be owned by the corporations that have purchased the land and extracted the oil. But when large oil deposits were discovered on the north slope of Alaska in the 1980s, they took a different approach. The Alaska Constitution requires that state resources be managed for the benefit of its people. Consequently, the Alaska Permanent Fund Corporation annually returns income from the royalties generated by oil extraction to its citizens. These payments typically amount to $1,000 or so, paid to residents each year depending on the investment performance. These payments constitute a basic income guarantee, which, for a family of four, is substantial.

Outside of Alaska, however, what belongs to the people has mostly been given to private corporations at low or no cost for them to profit from. Consider fracking, now a major source of oil in the US. Tiny royalties are paid to the federal government for extracting oil through fracking on federal lands. Some royalties are paid to the landowners where the exploitation is done, but major frackers manage to evade them. Their strategies include complex accounting practices that deduct costs from royalties, misreporting production volumes, and adding hidden fees, among many others.

Henry George, a popular nineteenth-century political economist whose book *Progress and Poverty* sold millions of copies [301], reflected on major technological progress during that century, including the steam engine, power loom, and railroad. Pondering what the railroad would bring us, George predicted the rich would get richer and the poor would get poorer. In a July 4, 1877, oration he said, "No nation can be freer than its most oppressed, richer than its poorest, wiser than its most ignorant." He advocated for natural land everywhere to be regarded as a community resource, rather than as a private resource. Its increase in value should be recaptured as public revenue by the community, he suggested, eliminating the need for any taxes on productive enterprises. He argued for a single tax on land values to generate income that would stem rising inequality and thereby benefit society.

We value our income, so instead of taxing that, we might consider taxing unearned income, what economists call rents. When you sell a property you own, other than land, such as a stock or any valuable asset, you pay a tax on what are the capital gains, namely the increase in value between what you paid, the basis, and what you gained on the sale. But today's capital gains tax rate is considerably less than the rate of tax on income, a contradiction to Henry George's principle. One can avoid even that by bequeathing property to heirs who get a stepped-up basis. I learned much from attending Georgist conferences. We could update Henry George's idea of having only a single tax on capital gains (including land values), instead of taxing our earned income.

Consider Georgist land today to include the airwaves that allow radio and television broadcasts and the internet. This godlike technology was developed at government expense but, once it became profitable, was given away to industry. The broadcast media that evolved from this technology are based on an advertising business model to generate income. We, the people, are the product, sold to the advertisers by the producers of content. None of these profit-making ventures pay a royalty to us for using our airwaves. These airwaves are sold to big business to watch over us through surveillance capitalism or technofeudalism [276]. Instead of land ownership being the key source of power (as in feudalism), technofeudalism vests control over digital infrastructure, data, and online platforms to grant dominant tech companies near-monopolistic power that resides in the cloud; in other words, they are cloudalists. Users, workers, and even smaller businesses become dependent on these platforms, much like serfs in feudal times who relied on lords for access to land and protection. Its origins spring from governments funding basic research.

Vast research sums are spent by the government to produce other technical innovations. The ENIAC, or Electronic Numerical Integrator And Computer, was created by the US government during World War II. The government funded various improvements and subsidized further development to private industries such as International Business Machines Corporation (IBM) and Control Data before it became profitable. By the late 1970s, computers had become profitable, so the celestial technology, advanced at US government expense, was given away to private industry to become quite lucrative. This represents American-style capitalism with strong government technology development subsidies. Consider Apple and PCs today. Even our tiny smart devices carry more computing power than what got us to the Moon in 1969 – and virtually everyone has at least one such device.

The internet originated through the Defense Advanced Research Projects Agency (DARPA), again paid for by the public through taxation. Once profitable, this divine technology was given away free, and has produced today's tech giants, including Amazon, Apple, Google, Meta (Facebook), and Microsoft. Their income now comes from technofeudalism-generated cloud rent. We are sold to the cloudalists!

The passenger airplane is the outcome of another government-funded initiative, when we developed bombers to use in wars. Through our taxes, we paid for initial design and subsequent improvements for them to become lethal weapons. Boeing and other aircraft manufacturers used this technology without paying royalties to us and made huge profits with the passenger airplanes they produced.

With a small royalty fee paid to the citizens who funded the development of these beatific technologies, we could use those resources to lessen economic inequality and thereby improve our health.

Today's subsidies are another major force that doesn't serve our health.

GOVERNMENT SUBSIDIES TODAY

Corporations have a disproportionate role in shaping public policy. Mergers have led to only a few companies controlling much of the processed food industry. Four supermarket chains predominate in a quasi-monopoly, exerting great pressure on lawmakers to pass laws favoring industry.

Recall our government budget, where huge sums are spent on the military and considerably lesser discretionary amounts on what might or might not benefit our health. In 2020, subsidies were paid to tobacco farmers who produce a lethal but legal substance that sickens us. Benefits to oil companies are in the order of tens of billions of dollars annually, and are much more than those given to renewable energy. Worldwide fossil fuel subsidies add up to more than $5 trillion out of a global gross domestic product (GDP) total of over $100 trillion. These handouts massively favor the economic elite. We are harming even the elite through the massive transfer of wealth via these archaic institutions by making their lives shorter and sicker.

Ralph Estes, a conservative accountant and professor at American University, tallied the cost to the public of private US corporations as $2.6 trillion in 1991 [302]. He argued that without such help they would have gone out of business.

Farm subsidies, beginning after the Great Depression, today promote corn growth, the leading crop in the US. We get high-fructose corn syrup used in processed foods that harm us. Other supports are for soy, wheat, and rice. Almost no subsidies are for healthy fruits or vegetables. Cargill, headquartered in Minnesota, but incorporated in Delaware (the corporate tax haven), is the largest privately held US corporation and enjoys huge government subsidies.

These are collective actions that harm our health. What can an individual do outside of this process?

INDIVIDUAL ACTIONS: MOVING TO A HEALTHIER PLACE?

Does it make sense to pack up and go somewhere else to live a healthier life? There are no studies of the health benefits to Americans of moving to a healthier nation. What if you live in a less healthy part of the United States and move to a healthier county or state? One thorough long-term randomized study ("Moving to Opportunity") looked at families relocating from neighborhoods with extreme poverty to less deprived areas [303]. Economic self-sufficiency did not improve for them, but their well-being did. Benefits included reduced extreme obesity, less diabetes, and improved mental health.

Unfortunately, if you move from a healthier country, such as Japan, to the United States, your health will become worse than if you had not resettled [304]. Japanese culture is good for health, especially given their sense of social support, discussed in Chapter 3.

Some immigrating to the US, however, such as people who migrate from Mexico, see their health improve. The epidemiological or Hispanic paradox finds that those coming from less healthy countries in Latin America do have lower mortality after they move here. However the advantage diminishes with the amount of time the immigrant stays. Reasons postulated include the healthy migrant effect (those who come are healthier than others left behind) and the salmon hypothesis (old people go home to die). But the social support that Latinx provide to friends and family, which is ingrained in their culture, best explains the finding [305]. This healthy immigrant paradox may be true for those coming from African nations too. Such an effect improves health through immigration. But "unhealthy assimilation" occurs within a generation, and then across subsequent generations as people encounter and begin to succumb to American individualism. But having more immigration to the US could result in overall health improvements by Americans adopting our newcomers' sense of social support.

Our high level of income inequality produces unfavorable outcomes for us all. Across America we find increased residential income segregation as the rich cluster in gated communities and the poor live in ghettos. America has the most poverty of all rich nations, so housing segregation, as well as racial segregation, has not improved. Housing insecurity, together with the large population of unhoused, is a major health problem in the US.

Upward mobility is part of the "American Dream," so people may find ways to move out of a poorer neighborhood by various means, including taking out loans they may not be able to pay. This could compound their economic issues and make them feel worse.

What are some lessons from these studies? I tell people that if they want to smoke cigarettes they should arrange to be born in Japan! If you are very poor and live in a disadvantaged neighborhood, moving to a better place may improve your health a little. The benefits of moving will be better for those who are younger. But your best bet is if you move before being conceived! You should not be conceived by poor parents, nor grow up in poverty. Unfortunately, almost none of this advice is practical for individuals. The United States needs to dismantle its disadvantaged neighborhoods and cities and consider opening US borders to more immigrants, not fewer. That could improve the overall health status of the country, not only because having healthier people here would raise our life expectancy, but also because some of the salutary social factors might rub off on the rest of us.

For this to happen, however, our society needs to put structures in place to generate good health.

What about individual actions of the sort we are constantly exposed to?

OTHER INDIVIDUAL ACTIONS REGARDING YOUR HEALTH

Your income or wealth likely puts you in the top 10% or below. No matter where you stand, the most important task is to collapse the gap and use the proceeds to support early life and decrease the record levels of poverty in the US.

With fear of the mass shootings in the United States, sales of bullet-proof vests and backpacks are soaring, which represents a form of body armor different from that of obesity. Should you send your student to school with such a backpack and instructions to duck and hold the backpack in front of you for protection? Consider the societal reasons for mass shootings, namely income inequality and the presence of high incomes [172]. A parent purchasing a bulletproof backpack for a child's use at school admits failure to consider the upstream determinants of health in the US.

This book is not an advice or self-help manual for what you should do as an individual to be healthy. It is a society-help guidebook. However, some personal advice follows.

Eat healthy foods; avoid known bad behaviors; get regular exercise; and seek appropriate medical care when needed.

The American medical care system performs poorly among rich countries in reducing avoidable deaths for conditions that medical care can treat effectively. We all get sick and seek healthcare. Navigating to get the best such care is a challenge. Ask appropriate questions of caregivers to gauge their efficacy. Point out to them how poorly America does in providing healthcare. Recognize clinicism (i.e. health is a result of personal behaviors and medical care), which is a distraction from what really matters [306]. Be confident that the care you are receiving is beneficial care.

Being involved in a community and having social support are necessary for health. Do everything you can to seek out others near you for support when needed and for friendship generally. Make this social interaction face to face and not virtual. Limit your use of smart devices when they interfere with such contact. Avoid multitasking when you're interacting with others. Instead carve out the time to work together.

The next chapter will lay out what needs to be done to not be born sick and die young. But first, we need to know, what changes policy in the United States?

WHAT CHANGES US POLICY

University of Michigan political scientist John Kingdon, studying policy changes in the United States, found three factors were necessary for the success of a policy change [307]. The first required nationwide attention to the problem. Next, there had to be specific policy solutions. While this seems enough to produce the needed change in other countries, the US requires a third ingredient – a policy window for the *transformation*. In 1911, the Triangle Shirtwaist Factory burned down, killing 146 workers, mostly women. Locked inside the overcrowded, unsafe, building, workers leapt to their deaths to avoid the fire. The horrific nature of their deaths, and the revelation of their working conditions, led to workplace safety regulations and gave renewed power to the labor movement. Russia launched Sputnik in 1957; that achievement led to a policy window spurring our goal of landing a human on the moon by the end of the next decade. And the September 11, 2001, terrorist attacks led to passage of the Patriot Act with all its surveillance mechanisms and subsequent invasions of Afghanistan and Iraq. Not all change is constructive.

Following Kingdon's model, we first need to draw attention to the problem and present specific policy solutions, which is the topic of the next chapter.

CHAPTER TEN

Toward a Healthy United States of America

If you have come here to help me, you are wasting your time . . . but if you have come because your liberation is bound up with mine, then let us work together.

Lilla Watson

America faces a calamity. The storming of the Capitol on January 6, 2021, is a major sign of discord. Mass shootings are so common they no longer make headlines. A huge political division distracts people from what is going on by "divide and conquer" strategies, and the public has become increasingly politically polarized. We have become poorer as our quality of life has declined. Will this country continue its health decline as Russia did after the 1991 breakup of the USSR? Or will we come to our senses?

Walt Kelly's character Pogo, in a 1971 Earth Day cartoon, surveyed the dumped garbage in the swamp, and said: "Yes son, we have met the enemy, and he is us." To defeat the enemy, we must be ready when the crisis or shock occurs, the event that is the window of opportunity that Kingdon's analysis says is required to ignite change [308].

FROM TRANSFORMATIVE EVENT TO EFFECTIVE SOLUTIONS

That event could be an unexpected election outcome; a major invention that changes our lives; the effects of a major storm, fire, or earthquake; a human-caused disaster; or some other calamity. But before Kingdon's political window opens, we must be ready by having raised awareness of the problem, which is our declining health, as well as a consensus on proposed solutions, namely decreasing inequality through increased taxation and supporting early life. Today, people's lives are so stressed that they feel pessimistic about making meaningful change. Optimism, a Paleolithic emotion, can lead others to think positively. Most Americans would like to have paid parental leave, free or very low-cost childcare and preschool, and accessible higher education. But these are unlikely with current US capitalism. Frame an effective solution in your own words to present to anyone you engage in discussion – and work for legislative change in the political system.

But if all this sounds too daunting, what else might you consider?

STATE OF THE UNION

The State of the Union address is required by the US Constitution to inform the Congress. The typical phrase used is that the state of the union is strong. Only one president, Gerald Ford in 1975, said, "the state of the union is not good." This came in the wake of the Watergate scandal that led to President Nixon's resignation after the failed US invasion of Vietnam. The phrase that would most honestly describe the state of our union should be along the lines of, "the state of the union is not healthy."

The address should make comparisons with other unions. The president would report that, this year, US life expectancy did not improve in contrast that of to other rich unions, but fell to where it was 28 years ago. They would go on to say that this is worrisome since something similar happened in Russia 34 years ago after the fall of the Soviet Union. They could say that those who are richer are not as healthy as those who are less rich in many other nations. They could say that, although we are chasing happiness, attaining it is more elusive than before.

Countries have goals, such as the US announced in the 1960s when it declared we would land a man on the Moon by the end of the 1960s. The president could lay out a national goal that we would once again be among the healthiest nations as we once were in the early 1950s. That is ludicrous you say. It would be like the president shooting themself in the foot. Yet in 2010 a task force of the Australian government did just that when it announced a goal to become the world's healthiest nation and beat out Japan [309]. It even laid out a plan to accomplish this.

Such a jolt would begin the process of rehealing America. What other novel ideas might we consider to put Kingdon's ideas into practice?

RESTRUCTURING SOCIETY

We need a basic rethinking of society's purpose and who is best served. Harvard philosopher John Rawls suggested the veil of ignorance. How would you design a society not knowing how you will end up? Starting from scratch, how would you organize the nation? Recognizing the inequities in society and who prospers from them, Rawls suggested that they should benefit those who are worst off [310]. Our society today is vastly different from the one Rawls promoted though, because we mostly support the most advantaged. What are additional perspectives?

Adapt the Swiss cheese model to attain better health. The cheese holes are created by a bacterium producing carbon dioxide that leaves bubbles or holes when the cheese cures. When you pile slices of Swiss cheese from different batches on top of one another, the holes will not line up. You won't be able to see through any one hole. With only one layer of our metaphorical Swiss cheese, a cavity can let something through that makes our health worse. Any individual effort would have flaws or holes. But with enough layers, it would be impossible for the illness-producing toxin to penetrate. Each layer in the model can have a different purpose [311]. What might these layers represent in our effort to improve US health?

One layer is an effective government that supports early life through paid parental leave, free or low-cost childcare, eradication of child poverty, and free education, among things – which all cost money. Several layers would raise taxes on the rich to pay for these initiatives. One such layer would be a progressive income tax. Another would be a substantial wealth tax. With enough of these layers, there is no way for poor health to penetrate.

The New Deal described earlier had many cheese layers superimposed to prevent those most impacted by the Great Depression from falling into the bottomless poverty pit. Layers included social security, high income taxes, and job programs. The government spent tax revenue to support the public who were hard hit by the economic depression. We know how to make a country healthy. We also did it in Japan after World War II.

Despite the devastation the US wrought on Japan during World War II, America helped make Japan the world's healthiest nation, as discussed in Chapter 5. General Douglas MacArthur's policies of demilitarization, democratization, and decentralization, the three Ds that were enshrined in the constitution written for them, resulted in the most rapid improvement ever in health. This medicine, rapidly decreasing economic inequality, is tested and effective. We could take the same medicine or ask Japan to give it to us. All that needs to be done is to persuade "we the people" to take this miracle drug! Paradoxically, in the United States today, we are doing the converse, namely increasing our military might, diverting to rule by plutocrats, and centralizing wealth among the few. How to stop this and focus on the real issue?

PERSUADING OTHERS

We must build a movement around achieving better health. If the gap in health outcomes both within the United States and around the world were to diminish significantly, most other dysfunctional aspects of society would improve. Narrowing the global gap between the best health and the poorest health among nations would improve the environment, begin to address global warming, decrease violence and war, and set the planet on the path for a sustainable future.

Anand Giridharadas presents useful methods [312]. Converse and canvas. Don't water things down, as you won't persuade people through dilution. Thin gruel doesn't taste very good. He advises us to make big and bold demands, and to stick to them. Revisit someone you talked to about your concepts. Form coalitions that are like families. A family that doesn't fight at home is in trouble. But be careful how you fight. Anger is needed for survival, but contempt is fatal to a relationship. There is much scorn and dismissal on so many social media platforms today. Know when to air things, but don't defer to keep the peace. Know your circles of influence, but recognize that other people will see the problem differently. Don't descend into fear, scapegoating, and xenophobia. Instead ask, "Have you considered this study?" This approach counters the right's lie- and hate-spewing demagogues. They take the hammer of rampant disinformation and beat people with it. Many have their own "alternative" facts in our post-truth world. Even the idea that the Sun orbits the Earth has a ring of truthiness to those who see themselves at the center of the universe.

The right uses the power of the corporate media, which won't call out fascism (i.e. decaying capitalism), to manage perception. The power of the right advantages only the top 1%, those who already have too much.

The appeal to emotions of those on the right has made the right very successful, as they resort to fearmongering over the latest threat to their way of life by provoking emotions through warnings of a new red scare with communists infiltrating our society, immigrant hoards rushing our borders, or "woke" ideology sexualizing our children. Triggering emotions works – something the advertising industry recognized half a century ago when it shifted from commercials that focused on the product and its attributes to announcements that need not show or discuss the product at all – but focus, instead, on the feelings the product will produce in you, while associating that emotion with their brand. Want to feel like you've achieved something? Wear Nikes. Want to be happy? Drink Coca-Cola. Want to feel confident? Try a new deodorant, or menstrual pad, or medicine. Whatever the product is, throw in a dog, cat, or cute baby, and the viewer will associate that product with positive emotions. As the fictional ad executive Don Draper says in the series *Mad Men*, "Advertising is based on one thing: happiness. And you know what happiness is? The smell of a new car." Or as expressed in a full-page Macy's ad for Ralph Lauren that ran in *The New York Times*, "What makes you happy? Luxury every day." If only our health weren't such an elusive luxury.

Appealing to emotions has always moved people. Yet the left has not been very successful in presenting what actions and policies are needed for economic and political justice, because their arguments appeal to logic. The left needs to play to emotions and feelings, including fear and anxiety, if it wants to reach a wider audience.

Be anxious about not being healthy. Be aware of what others care about and speak to that. Many young people want to be influencers. If you want to influence the conversation, figure out what influencers do and become one yourself. Find out what people care about and speak to that.

Inundating people with facts and statistics doesn't work. Mother Teresa said, "If I look at the mass I will never act. If I look at the one, I will." Mass murders, genocides, and other mass trauma have a psychic numbing effect. They depict humans with their tears dried off and don't trigger emotions. We react to a human-interest story with tear-faced emojis, but not to a media report with millions of deaths. Ask someone if they know two Americans under age 65 who died. Point out that if they had lived in Australia, Canada, Germany, Japan, or Portugal, only one would have died [8].

What is the relationship between the number of lives and the value of saving one? With our Paleolithic emotions, we experienced few lives lost in the forager-hunter era. We could feel the loss. With today's "God-given" technology, we have come to accept that, with so many lives lost, one more doesn't matter. This is the uppermost problem in dealing with America's health decline. It is too gargantuan for a reasoned response. We have to change the paradigm surrounding health and healthcare.

Healthcare access is desired in America. But we are loath to change our broken medical care system. When the Obama administration presented the American Affordable Care Act (ACA), the right quickly branded it, "Obamacare." Predictably, conservatives rejected the plan – but when asked if they supported the ACA, the majority of those who rejected "Obamacare" indicated that they fully supported the ACA!

The language framing a problem shapes how it's perceived. Present the ideal of universal healthcare to those who have resisted the concept, but in order for it to not be considered as a socialist plot, call it the public option. Point out that the healthcare *insurance* system is a ruling force on Americans who don't like to be ruled by others. When someone protests that they don't want their taxes going up to pay for it, tell them the insurance premiums they're paying are a hidden tax, one that will go down, or be eliminated altogether, so they'll bring home more money. Remind them as well that their employer keeps their wages down, because they're paying into this hidden tax in the form of employer-paid contributions to that premium. When they no longer have to pay that premium, they can pay higher wages. Frame Medicare for all as an American ideal rather than a governmental program, since so many people here have embraced Ronald Reagan's declaration and now believe that government remains the problem.

Stock up on perspectives of economic inequality such as presented in the weekly online newsletter from inequality.org. It presents pictures to sway emotions, graphical elements, and much food for thought.

Be comfortable talking about politics, beginning with your friends and family and extending to the public arena. Americans tend to avoid discussing politics, especially among those they are not close to.

Focus on the world we want rather than what we oppose in the world that we have. Rather than blaming the victims of unchecked disinformation, we should enlist them to treat our malignancy. Your actions may influence people more than your words. Make yourself available for discussions with others. Answer inquiries from people who disagree with you. You may find that naysayers are not fervently committed to their points of view. In not being self-defeating, you may find both of you can prosper from a conversation that is not one-sided by focusing only on the world you desire. Say what you are for, but affirm what others say while you talk in a nonthreatening fashion. Look at the big picture.

CREATING NATIONWIDE ATTENTION

How can we create awareness of the problem? People's attention spans are short, so to draw attention to the problem; you must be quick and your efforts effective. Start by learning some one-liners to spark interest. I sometimes call them killer facts! Consider using mine:

- Americans are dead first. Something that is a killer fact!
- Inequality kills.
- You cannot buy health; it is not for sale.
- Do you want health or healthcare?
- Instead of teaching the facts of life, we must teach the facts of death.
- We must love one another or die.
- America is a no-vacation nation.
- Americans have the right to life, but it is only a short one.
- The right to liberty is an illusion given that we house a quarter of the world's prisoners.
- We are only allowed to pursue happiness, not to attain it.
- Sixty-three percent of all statistics are made up on the spot. (Using this phrase makes you stand out in the eyes of some folk who may want to listen more.)
- All generalizations are false.
- I have an X chromosome deficiency disorder, pointing out my maleness.
- On average, we have one breast and one testicle. This fact shows how averages can be misleading.
- As you go from the erection to the resurrection, the first 1,000 days after conception matter the most for your health.
- What is the most common sexually transmitted infection? Life! You are all here because your father's sperm infected or fertilized your mother's ovum

that she produced when she was in your grandmother's womb. (That is a huge mouthful but contains many ideas presented in this book.)

- There are only two countries in the world that don't have a national policy to grant a working pregnant woman paid time off after she has her baby. One is the USA. The other is Papua New Guinea, half of a big island north of Australia.

Make up our own, and when you find a good one, please share it with me.

COMMUNICATION CHANNELS

Use the channels of communication available to you. There are limitless opportunities in the virtual realm.

For the last quarter century, I have incorporated student activism exercises in the university courses I have taught. My students are required to take the ideas presented in the classroom and broadcast them outside. Before COVID-19 these were in-person meetings planned in advance. With the pandemic they became virtual, where they have remained as the numbers they can reach are far greater. They are visionaries who are becoming student activists.

Inform your friends and followers on Facebook, Instagram, X (formerly Twitter), and TikTok. Recognize that social media has resulted in a huge communication transformation. People spend much more time on their devices than previously, so face-to-face and real-time conversations have become less common. This metamorphosis has increased isolation and loneliness with major consequences for mental health. The UK government recognized this by creating a "Minister for Loneliness." We have entered an age of insecurity and of rage with the loss of many genuine conversations with one another, whether in the home, at work, or at play. We need to resurrect that art of real-time communication. Opportunities abound to practice this amongst friends, family, and coworkers, as well as with strangers in various venues. I tell my students to enhance their population health conversation skills when they get a marketing phone call that is being recorded for quality assurance purposes. The caller won't hang up and you can practice engaging them in fruitful discussion.

OTHER IDEAS

Ask questions in a way that seeks to understand. "Why do you think your health is under your own control?" Don't be judgmental in the response you get. If you put someone down for their beliefs, there is little hope in changing them.

Create your own group that deals with the book's issues. I started the Population Health Forum (PHF) in Seattle, a voluntary organization, almost three decades ago. We had no budget so did not have to spend time fundraising. Besides holding regular meetings discussing US health issues, we have created a website as a useful repository, and have developed and implemented school classes on population health, among many activities.

Consider hosting a group event where this book's ideas are discussed. One example the PHF used is having an event with an informational speaker such as Richard Wilkinson. Beforehand, we scheduled subsequent events at local libraries and produced flyers announcing the events, which were put on the audience seats. Our forum then continued discussions at these events.

New resources can aid discussion. One is the interactive data visualization website produced by our national Centers for Disease Control and Prevention at www.cdc.gov/nchs/data-visualization/life-expectancy/. It used to publish maps of life expectancies for US states as well as counties, and even census tracts for the period 2010–2015. The current administration has removed that source. In the future it may return, allowing you to produce such a map and muse about the huge differences (up to 40 years) in lifespan over small areas. When speaking at a specific place in the United States, I present such a regional map from the CDC to the audience depicting the worst health in red and the best in blue. They can identify these areas and typically see the socioeconomic gradient in action. Point out that there can't be differences in personal behaviors or medical care that can amount to those gigantic variations in health outcomes.

Remember the serenity prayer: God, grant me the serenity to accept the things I cannot change, the courage to change the things I can, and the wisdom to know the difference.

What are you going to do with your one and only precious life? Consider activism, taking direct action. What might that look like?

Wear your issues and values. In public I wear one of two baseball hats, both blue. One is lettered "Make America Equal Again" and the other "Make America Healthy Again." People notice and often remark that they like my hat. I don't wear T-shirts, because they don't have pockets for my pencil and notebook, without which I am naked. But lettered designs could be one of the lines above. Search the internet for activist T-shirts for striking designs such as "Destroy the patriarchy, not the planet," or "Think while it is still legal."

My bumper sticker reads, "Don't believe everything you think!"

Attend demonstrations and carry a sign, or when marching with others, a banner. At the November 1999 World Trade Organization (WTO) demonstrations in Seattle, I carried a sign that read "WTO makes us sick." I was approached by a local radio station to come and talk to their audience. Short cleverly worded signage attracts attention!

Consider addressing issues you face regularly in your work. As a teacher at the University of Washington, and in other organizations that I belong to, most events precede with a land acknowledgment. As part of colonizing the United States, the land was seized from the local inhabitants, the Indigenous, First Nations, natives, or so-called American Indians, without any recompense. The land acknowledgment, a condensed version along the lines of "We occupy lands surrounding the Salish Sea that were previously home to many tribes that we colonized and tried to decimate," has become more routine in some settings than singing the national anthem or any other invocation. After it is voiced, nothing is done. Why not add a US poor health status acknowledgment? Something along the lines of "We live in a country that is less healthy than all the other rich nations and a considerable number of poor ones."

An important way that educational institutions can cover various topics is to have them be on various required examinations. Then schools will teach to the test. As an example, for public health schools, there is an accreditation body, Council on Education for Public Health (CEPH), which lays out criteria that a college or university must meet to claim this status. One of the current competencies is to look at "causes and trends of morbidity and mortality in the US or other community relevant to the school or program." That leaves almost all US schools of public health neglecting comparing American health with that of other nations. This can't be altered until 2026 or afterwards. I'm proposing that it be then amended to include "describing trends over the last half-century, as well as making comparisons with other nations." In addition, there are no similar examination topics for college students applying to medical school (Medical College Admission Test [MCAT]), nor for the exams of graduating medical students (United States Medical Licensing Examination [USMLE]), among many others in the healthcare realm. One could also have the SAT, used for college admission, cover US health status as depicted in this book. You readers who have the opportunity to set standards for the various tests American students undergo have a great opportunity here.

Some activists have spent time in jail and speak proudly of incarceration as a direct-action badge of courage.

Consider local organizations to join and work with. One national organization, Physicians for Social Responsibility (PSR), has state branches, such as Washington PSR (WPSR). Most members are not physicians. The PSR has been involved in winning two Nobel Prizes for its antinuclear work. The WPSR has an economic inequality health task force that holds regular meetings. We, the members, are health activists, empowered by compassion and undaunted by the odds.

People sleep, work, and socialize. We should have democracy in the workplace. Democracy grants "power to the people," a 1960s slogan. But in most typical capitalist workplace settings, we have no power to control what work is about, what is produced, and who benefits. If we did have power, we could structure a very different work environment. Democracy at Work (d@w) is a movement working toward that goal; visit its website, www.democracyatwork.info. Listen to the weekly broadcast Economic Update. The presenter, Richard D Wolff, an unusual academic economist with degrees from Harvard, Stanford, and Yale, has pointed out that since the 1970s US worker wages, adjusted for inflation, have not increased, while worker productivity has soared. Neoliberalism, reverting to nineteenth-century free-market capitalism, discussed in the previous chapter, brought about the divergence. I verified his ideas. Recall comparisons of the median two-parent, two-child family finances in 1970 and 2000. It is like putting a jigsaw puzzle together. The pieces all fit, and then you can show it to others. As work time increases, sleep and socialization have suffered.

THE PEOPLE UNITED

How can democracy happen at work? Worker-owned enterprises and cooperatives are one way. Requiring boards of directors of corporations to have substantial representation by their workers is another and is common in Germany. Scandinavian countries lean toward social democracies that have more ubiquitous people power.

Reform and strengthen labor unions. Elite forces have managed to successfully decimate organized labor. A resurgence today gives hope to worker power.

Support the Poor People's Campaign to support a living wage. A huge demonstration was proposed by Dr. Martin Luther King Jr. in 1968, but after he was assassinated, it never happened. That movement has been revived and is growing.

Today's Poor People's Campaign calls for a moral revival. Poverty kills, and yet, impoverished people don't vote. Impoverished and low-wage people make up 30% of the US electorate, and in battleground states they account for nearly 40%. One main reason they don't vote is that no politician speaks to their problems. None of the presidential debates addresses poverty, nor our declining health. The Poor People's Campaign seeks to change this by waking the sleeping giant, the poor and low-wage workers. We must protect and expand the right to vote by reinstating the key protections of the 1965 Voting Rights Act, which is being fiercely attacked today through antivoter measures. If we get poor and low-wage workers out to vote, health will improve for the rest of us.

Make cross-national comparisons. I carry a clipboard with comparison graphics. In discussing almost any issue, I want to know how other nations do. On the back of my clipboard is a biohazard symbol lettered: *Economic Inequality Is Hazardous to Our Health.* In face-to-face gatherings I may hold it up to my chest to display my issues. An activist friend has produced such lettered T-shirts, coasters, cups, and stickers for sale on the internet. This is an example of efforts by an introvert who won't speak out vocally at demonstrations.

Not everyone is swayed by visual information. Some may remember a striking graphic, such as the map of life expectancy in Chapter 3, but people are more likely to be impacted by stories.

We learn best from stories. I realized I was a socialist in 1974 by asking to be paid the same as my coworker who had no medical credentials. Keep track of such experiences. I keep a pencil and paper by my bed so ideas that drift in and out of my dreamscape can be written down and remembered. The same with my shirt pocket. Others will use their smartphones to capture thoughts. Whatever works. You never know when a creative thought will appear.

Keep records of your experiences and the stories they produce and organize them on your computer or device so that they can easily be searched when you need to look something up.

I'm a visual learner. I have over 18 gigabytes of slide files on my computer organized into different subject areas. One file is named Solutions. To prepare this chapter, I examined those images.

FINDING YOUR PATH

How to decide upon a cause to lend time/money to?

Such a decision, namely working with an organization, requires integrating your personal values with those of your family, friends, coworkers, and those whom you respect.

The key message of this book is that our health, that of all of us, including you the reader and me the author, is not very good if the standard is making comparisons with people in all the other rich countries and quite a few poorer ones. Key reasons presented are the American lack of support for early life and our high economic inequality.

Begin by reflecting on whether you believe these concepts by considering your personal experiences and those of others. Are they consistent with your values and beliefs? Recalling the downstream/upstream metaphor used by the Hawai'i State Department of Health, are you comfortable with politics as the most upstream factor impacting health? You may need to do more research to convince yourself.

Next ask yourself if you want your health, together with that of your children and grandchildren, to be as good as possible? Assuming you do, are you willing to accept that change has to occur nationally, rather than by dealing with individual behaviors?

As pointed out in previous chapters, national political changes happen slowly for the most part. Accepting that typically requires working together with others over considerable time. There are many organizations out there to contemplate joining if you don't create your own.

Which ones might be candidates? Begin by inventorying your resources, time, money, and skills. If you don't enjoy doing something, you won't do it for long. What skills can you bring to the efforts? I enjoy teaching, writing, and speaking, so have developed skills there. I'm not so good at organizing groups and being a leader.

Having determined your personal inventory, look at the myriad organizations out there. You may get many funding requests. Check out those groups. The easiest way is to look at their websites. What are they about? Their visions, values, strategies? What can you discover about their staff and leaders? What is their evidence base? Their financial structure? Do they mostly fundraise or direct more efforts to action and activism? How do they measure progress or success? How much transparency do they have? What is their culture? Are they insensitive to parts of your value system that are important to you?

Search the internet for other groups.

Many organizations produce publications. Check them out and use Google Scholar to find how others cite these publications and what they say about them. Search on social media for reactions as well.

Make contact with someone in that organization and gauge the interaction. Volunteer your time for some event to gain experience in how they operate. Engage with others in that group. Perhaps key individuals there have discussions you can access on YouTube. I find this a very valuable way to get to know such principals in an organization.

If you primarily plan to contribute time or money, is this mostly to cover administrative costs or for working toward real change?

Although this process may take considerable time, you will get a sense of whether or not this is meaningful for you or the right fit for you.

WORKING TOGETHER

One person can't do much, so don't be one person. The African proverb says, "If you want to go fast, go alone. If you want to go far, go together." Make coalitions to work together. What is the work that must be done? We need to develop a force to produce creative maladjustment in society.

This requires much more than hope for change; it requires a strategy to tackle the enormous inequality in America and the resulting lack of attention to what produces good health. Once people recognize that they die first, namely they don't live the longer, healthier lives that people in other nations do, we must change the status quo and decrease inequality, and use the proceeds to support early life. Merely voting in today's elections won't do much. Large public support for improving health through massive demonstrations, and a far-reaching media campaign, can result in profound changes, such as the demonstrations that ended the US invasion of Vietnam. Massive social movements are the forces we need now.

I've presented the big picture of what produces health in a society together with steps to get the US moving in the direction of better health improvements. The required changes are systemic and revolutionary. They also challenge capitalism in today's neoliberal society. To convince those who have too much that their abundance is limiting how healthy they are today, and that their health and that of their children and grandchildren would be better by their being less rich, is the watershed moment.

Consider some wise words from others. Ghandi said, "First they ignore you, then they laugh at you, then they fight you, then you win." From Nelson Mandela: "It always seems impossible until it is done." And Angela Davis said, "I am no longer accepting the things I cannot change; I'm changing the things I cannot accept."

There is hope. Action and activism are the antidote to despair. Act now.

Epilogue

The world is facing new turmoil as this book goes into production in 2025. The United States is now seen as one of the countries supporting strongman governments acting above the rule of law. The fact that popular support has arisen for such seemingly undemocratic choices speaks to a more basic, perhaps universal, cause. I believe the increasing economic inequality within so many nations, which has surged in the last few decades, is the main culprit. Public support for demagogues appears highest where health is declining, which is catalyzed by rising inequity. Power in the US is becoming more concentrated, and there seems to be no way to counter that phenomenon.

President Trump has used questionably legal executive orders to dismantle parts of the government in the name of increasing efficiency. His appointments to major federal departments are minions who pledge loyalty to him and espouse draconian policies. Support for decreasing inequality and policies that foster a healthy early life are casualties of Trump's and Elon Musk's efforts. Income and wealth inequality will soar, with likely increases in mortality levels. Americans yet to be conceived or in the stages of early life will face challenges unseen in the last half-century.

Repercussions in other parts of the world from the suspension of US foreign aid are already apparent. Tariff policies will likely foster economic conflicts and increase the threat of nuclear war. Global warming will accelerate human havoc.

What will get us out of this pandemonium? Historically, it has been world wars. The most recent one resulted in the United States dropping two atomic bombs on Japan, the only time such power has ever been unleashed on a nation. The failure of diplomacy in conflicts today is very worrisome. The US empire is in decline, while China's is ascending and may be on the verge of overtaking America's. The Cold War resulting from the USSR's threat to American hegemony evaporated with the Soviet Union, but we are in another cold war that threatens to turn hot.

Humans want to be healthy, an aim that is increasingly elusive. Seeking to accomplish that goal requires intervening at the national level or beyond. Given enough time and effort, there is no biological reason that any nation cannot be as healthy as the healthiest. However, current trends are moving us in the opposite direction.

What is to be done? Creating awareness is the first step. Use the concepts in Chapter 10 to build people power. Together we can weather this storm and come out stronger.

About the Author

Stephen Bezruchka AM, MD, MPH has worked in health and healthcare for over 50 years. A graduate of Stanford Medical School, with a public health degree from Johns Hopkins University, his career began by helping set up a community health project in a Himalayan valley a week's walk from the road in Nepal (for the full story, see the book *Far From the Road: A Community Health Project in the Himalayas*, www.farfromtheroad.com). He later set up a remote district hospital there as a teaching hospital for Nepali doctors, whom he supervised. He spent over 30 years practicing as an emergency physician in the United States. He studied pure mathematics at Harvard, attaining a master's degree, before pursuing medicine. This instilled a desire to understand the production of health in populations. He joined the faculty of the School of Public Health at the University of Washington in 1994 and taught courses looking at the country as the "patient." His previous books are *Trekking in Nepal: A Traveler's Guide*, *Nepali for Trekkers*, *The Pocket Doctor: A Passport to Healthy Travel*, *Altitude Illness: Prevention and Treatment*, and *Inequality Kills Us All: COVID-19's Health Lessons for the World*. He can be contacted through his website: http://stephenbezruchka.com.

References

1. Prasad VK, Cifu AS. *Ending Medical Reversal: Improving Outcomes, Saving Lives.* Baltimore: Johns Hopkins University Press; 2015.

2. Avendano M, Glymour MM, Banks J, Mackenbach JP. Health disadvantage in US adults aged 50 to 74 years: A comparison of the health of rich and poor Americans with that of Europeans. *American Journal of Public Health.* 2009;**99**(3):540–8.

3. Banks J, Marmot M, Oldfield Z, Smith JP. Disease and disadvantage in the United States and in England. *JAMA.* 2006;**295**(17):2037–45.

4. Machado S, Kyriopoulos I, Orav EJ, Papanicolas I. Association between wealth and mortality in the United States and Europe. *New England Journal of Medicine.* 2025;**392**(13):1310–1319.

5. Emanuel EJ, Gudbranson E, Van Parys J, Gørtz M, Helgeland J, Skinner J. Comparing health outcomes of privileged US citizens with those of average residents of other developed countries. *JAMA Internal Medicine.* 2021;**181**(3):339–44.

6. Kochanek KD, Murphy SL, Xu JQ, Arias E. *Mortality in the United States, 2022. NCHS Data Brief, No. 492.* Hyattsville: National Center for Health Statistics; 2024.

7. Mokdad AH, Murray CJL. Reversing the decline of health in the USA: A call to action. *The Lancet.* 2024;**404**(10469):2392–4.

8. Bor J, Stokes AC, Raifman J, Venkataramani A, Bassett MT, Himmelstein D, et al. Missing Americans: Early death in the United States – 1933–2021. *PNAS Nexus.* 2023;**2**(6):1–13.

9. Cutler D, Miller G. The role of public health improvements in health advances: The twentieth-century United States. *Demography.* 2005;**42**(1):1–22.

10. Komlos J, Baur M. From the tallest to (one of) the fattest: The enigmatic fate of the American population in the 20th century. *Economics and Human Biology.* 2004;**2**: 57–74.

11. Woolf SH. Falling behind: The growing gap in life expectancy between the United States and other countries, 1933–2021. *American Journal of Public Health.* 2023;**113**(9):970–80.

12. Kuznets S. Economic growth and income inequality. *American Economic Review.* 1955;**45**(1):17–26.

13. Emanuel EJ. Why I hope to die at 75. *The Atlantic.* October 2014.

14. Helliwell JF, Layard R, Sachs J, De Neve J-E, Aknin LB, Wang S, eds. World Happiness Report 2024. Oxford: University of Oxford: Wellbeing Research Centre; 2024.

15. Lane RE. *The Loss of Happiness in Market Democracies.* New Haven: Yale University Press; 2000.

16. Makary MA, Daniel M. Medical Error – The third leading cause of death in the US. *BMJ.* 2016;**353**:i2139.

17. Anderson I. Hospital errors are number three killer in Australia. *New Scientist.* 1995;**146**:5.

18. Cunningham SA, Mitchell K, Narayan KM, Yusuf S. Doctors' strikes and mortality: A review. *Social Science & Medicine.* 2008;**67** (11):1784–8.

19. McClelland CE. *Queen of the Professions: The Rise and Decline of Medical Prestige and Power in America.* Lanham: Rowman & Littlefield; 2014.

20. Mintzes B. Advertising of prescription-only medicines to the public: Does evidence of benefit counterbalance harm? *Annual Review of Public Health.* 2012;**33**(1):259–77.

21. Jeurissen PPT, Kruse FM, Busse R, Himmelstein DU, Mossialos E, Woolhandler S. For-profit hospitals have thrived because of generous public reimbursement schemes, not greater efficiency: A multi-country case study. *International Journal of Health Services.* 2020;**51**(1):67–89.

22. Finkelstein A, McKnight R. What did Medicare do? The initial impact of Medicare on mortality and out of pocket medical spending. *Journal of Public Economics.* 2008;**92**(7):1644–68.

23. Hansen MR, Hróbjartsson A, Pottegård A, Damkier P, Larsen KS, Madsen KG, et al. Postponement of death by statin use: a systematic review and meta-analysis of randomized clinical trials. *Journal of General Internal Medicine.* 2019;**34**(8):1607–14.

24. Hansen MR, Hróbjartsson A, Videbæk L, Ennis ZN, Pareek M, Paulsen NH, et al. Postponement of death by pharmacological heart failure treatment: A meta-analysis of randomized clinical trials. *The American Journal of Medicine.* 2020;**133**(6):e280–9.

25. National Clinical Care Commission. *Report to Congress on Leveraging Federal Programs to Prevent and Control Diabetes and Its Complications.* Washington, DC: Office of Disease Prevention and Health Promotion; 2021.

26. Mayer-Davis EJ, Lawrence JM, Dabelea D, Divers J, Isom S, Dolan L, et al. Incidence trends of type 1 and type 2 diabetes among youths, 2002–2012. *New England Journal of Medicine.* 2017;**376**(15):1419–29.

27. Roseboom T, de Rooij S, Painter R. The Dutch famine and its long-term consequences for adult health. *Early Human Development.* 2006;**82**(8):485–91.

28. Mi D, Fang H, Zhao Y, Zhong L. Birth weight and type 2 diabetes: A meta-analysis. *Experimental and Therapeutic Medicine.* 2017;**14**(6):5313–20.

29. Basu S, Yoffe P, Hills N, Lustig RH. The relationship of sugar to population-level diabetes prevalence: An econometric analysis of repeated cross-sectional data. *PLOS ONE.* 2013;**8**(2):e57873.

30. Organisation for Economic Co-operation and Development (OECD). *Health at a Glance 2017: OECD Indicators.* Paris: OECD; 2017.

31. Kaplan RM, Milstein A. Contributions of health care to longevity: A review of 4 estimation methods. *Annals of Family Medicine.* 2019;**17**:267–72.

32. Abdalla SM, Hernandez M, Koya SF, Rosenberg SB, Robbins G, Magana L, et al. What matters for health? Public views from eight countries. *BMJ Global Health.* 2022;**7**(6):e008858.

33. Schneider EC, Shah A, Doty MM, Tikkanen R, Fields K, Williams II RD. *Mirror, Mirror 2021 – Reflecting Poorly: Health Care in the US Compared to Other High-Income Countries.* New York: The Commonwealth Fund; 2021.

34. Roos NP, Brownell M, Menec V. Universal medical care and health inequalities: right objectives, insufficient tools. In: Heymann J, Hertzman C, Barer ML, Evans RG, eds. *Healthier Societies: From Analysis to Action.* New York: Oxford University Press; 2006. pp. 107–31.

35. Nussbaum MC. Capabilities as fundamental entitlements: Sen and social justice. *Feminist Economics.* 2003;**9**(2):33–59.

36. Singh TP, Gauvreau K, Bastardi HJ, Blume ED, Mayer JE. Socioeconomic position and graft failure in pediatric heart transplant recipients. *Circulation: Heart Failure.* 2009;**2**(3):160–5.

37. Singh TP, Blume ED, Naftel DC, Foushee MT, Kirklin JK, Addonizio L, et al. Association of race and socioeconomic position with outcomes in pediatric heart transplant recipients. *American Journal of Transplantation.* 2010;**10**(9):2116–23.

38. DePasquale EC, Kobashigawa JA. Socioeconomic disparities in heart transplantation. *Circulation: Cardiovascular Quality and Outcomes.* 2016;**9**(6):693–4.

39. Basu S, Berkowitz SA, Phillips RL, Bitton A, Landon BE, Phillips RS. Association of primary care physician supply with population mortality in the United States, 2005–2015. *JAMA Internal Medicine.* 2019;**179**(4):506–14.

40. Bodenheimer T. Revitalizing primary care, part 1: Root causes of primary care's problems. *The Annals of Family Medicine.* 2022;**20**(5):464–8.

41. Bodenheimer T. Revitalizing primary care, part 2: Hopes for the future. *The Annals of Family Medicine.* 2022;**20**(5):469–78.

42. Michalec B, Cuddy MM, Price Y, Hafferty FW. US physician burnout and the proletarianization of US doctors: A theoretical reframing. *Social Science & Medicine.* 2024;**358**:117224.

43. Kalmoe MC, Chapman MB, Gold JA, Giedinghagen AM. Physician suicide: A call to action. *Missouri Medicine.* 2019;**116**(3):211–6.

44. Goozner M. Private equity takeovers are harming patients. *BMJ.* 2023;**382**:1396.

45. Victora CG, Bahl R, Barros AJD, França GVA, Horton S, Krasevec J, et al. Breastfeeding in the 21st century: Epidemiology, mechanisms, and lifelong effect. *The Lancet.* 2016;**387**(10017):475–90.

46. Miller CC. The world "has found a way to do this": The US lags on paid leave. *New York Times.* October 25, 2021. (Available from: www.nytimes.com/2021/10/25/upshot/paid-leave-democrats.html.)

47. Burtle A, Bezruchka S. Population health and paid parental leave: What the United States can learn from two decades of research. *Healthcare.* 2016;**4**(2):30.

48. Nandi A, Jahagirdar D, Dimitris MC, Labrecque JA, Strumpf EC, Kaufman JS, et al. The impact of parental and medical leave policies on socioeconomic and health outcomes in OECD countries: A systematic review of the empirical literature. *The Milbank Quarterly.* 2018;**96**(3):434–71.

49. Kaufman G. *Fixing Parental Leave: The Six Month Solution.* New York: New York University Press; 2020.

50. Lee RB, Daly RH, eds. *The Cambridge Encyclopedia of Hunters and Gatherers.* Cambridge: Cambridge University Press; 1999.

51. Pontzer H, Wood BM, Raichlen DA. Hunter-gatherers as models in public health. *Obesity Reviews.* 2018;**19**:24–35.

52. Flannery KV, Marcus J. *The Creation of Inequality: How our Prehistoric Ancestors Set the Stage for Monarchy, Slavery, and Empire.* Cambridge, MA, and London: Harvard University Press; 2012.

53. Larsen CS. The agricultural revolution as environmental catastrophe: Implications for health and lifestyle in the Holocene. *Quaternary International.* 2006;**150**(1):12–20.

54. Bezruchka S. Pathways to health and illness. In: Bryant T, ed. *Handbook on the Social Determinants of Health.* Cheltenham: Edward Elgar; 2025.

55. Wilson LG. The rise and fall of tuberculosis in Minnesota: The role of infection. *Bulletin of the History of Medicine.* 1992;**66**(1):16.

56. McKeown T. *The Role of Medicine: Dream, Mirage, or Nemesis.* Princeton: Princeton University Press; 1979.

57. Pobutsky A, Bradbury E, Wong Tomiyasu D. *Chronic Disease Disparities Report 2011: Social Determinants.* Honolulu: Hawai'i State Department of Health: Chronic Disease Management and Control Branch; 2011.

58. Lasswell HD. *Politics: Who Gets What, When, How.* New York: Meridian Books; 1958.

59. Pickett KE, Wilkinson RG. Income inequality and health: A causal review. *Social Science & Medicine.* 2015;**128**:316–26.

60. Kawachi I, Subramanian S. Income inequality. In: Berkman LF, Kawachi I, Glymour MM, eds. *Social Epidemiology.* New York: Oxford University Press; 2014. pp. 126–51.

61. Hall W. Social class and survival on the S.S. Titanic. *Social Science & Medicine.* 1986;**22**(6):687–90.

62. DeCelles KA, Norton MI. Physical and situational inequality on airplanes predicts air rage. *Proceedings of the National Academy of Sciences of the United States of America*. 2016;**113**(20):5588–91.

63. McLinton SS, Drury D, Masocha S, Savelsberg H, Martin L, Lushington K. "Air rage": A systematic review of research on disruptive airline passenger behaviour 1985–2020. *Journal of Airline and Airport Management*. 2020;**10**(1):31–49.

64. Piff PK, Stancato DM, Mendoza-Denton R, Keltner D, Coteb S. Higher social class predicts increased unethical behavior. *Proceedings of the National Academy of Sciences of the United States of America*. 2012;**109**(11):4086–91.

65. Sapolsky RM. *Behave: The Biology of Humans at Our Best and Worst.* New York: Penguin Press; 2017.

66. Brosnan SF, de Waal FBM. Evolution of responses to (un)fairness. *Science*. 2014;**346**(6207):1251776.

67. Riddell R, Ahmed N, Maitland A, Lawson M, Taneja A. *Inequality Inc. How Corporate Power Divides Our World and the Need for a New Era of Public Action.* Oxford: Oxfam International; 2024.

68. Kawachi I, Berkman L. Social capital, social cohesion, and health. In: Berkman LF, Kawachi I, Glymour MM, eds. *Social Epidemiology*. New York: Oxford University Press; 2014. pp. 290–319.

69. Ioannidis JA, Zonta F, Levitt M. Variability in excess deaths across countries with different vulnerability during 2020–2023. *Proceedings of the National Academy of Sciences of the United States of America*. 2023;**120**(49).

70. Cullen MR, Baiocchi M, Eggleston K, Loftus P, Fuchs V. The weaker sex? Vulnerable men and women's resilience to socio-economic disadvantage. *SSM – Population Health*. 2016;**2**: 512–24.

71. Rochelle TL, Yeung DKY, Bond MH, Li LMW. Predictors of the gender gap in life expectancy across 54 nations. *Psychology, Health & Medicine*. 2015;**20**(2):129–38.

72. Bezruchka S. *Inequality Kills Us All: COVID-19's Health Lessons for the World.* New York: Routledge; 2022.

73. Hofstede GH, Hofstede GJ. *Cultures and Organizations: Software of the Mind.* New York: McGraw-Hill; 2005.

74. Eckersley RM. Culture. In: Galea S, ed. *Macrosocial Determinants of Population Health.* New York: Springer; 2007. pp. 193–209.

75. Phelan JC, Link BG. Is racism a fundamental cause of inequalities in health? *Annual Review of Sociology*. 2015;**41**(1):311–30.

76. Jindal M, Trent M, Mistry KB. The intersection of race, racism, and child and adolescent health. *Pediatrics In Review*. 2022;**43**(8):415–25.

77. DeGruy J. *Post Traumatic Slave Syndrome: America's Legacy of Enduring Injury and Healing*. Milwaukie: Uptone Press; 2005.

78. Jasienska G. Low birth weight of contemporary African Americans: An intergenerational effect of slavery? *American Journal of Human Biology*. 2009;**21**(1):16–24.

79. Reverby S. *Examining Tuskegee: The Infamous Syphilis Study and Its Legacy*. Chapel Hill: University of North Carolina Press; 2009.

80. David RJ, Collins JW. Differing birth weight among infants of US-born Blacks, African-born Blacks, and US-born Whites. *New England Journal of Medicine*. 1997;**337**(17):1209–14.

81. Metzl J. *Dying of Whiteness: How the Politics of Racial Resentment Is Killing America's Heartland*. 1st ed. New York: Basic Books; 2019.

82. Katz DL, Meller S. Can we say what diet is best for health? *Annual Review of Public Health*. 2014;**35**(1):83–103.

83. Hauptman M, Niles JK, Gudin J, Kaufman HW. Individual- and community-level factors associated with detectable and elevated blood lead levels in US children results from a national clinical laboratory. *JAMA Pediatrics*. 2021;**175**(12):1252–60.

84. Vanderbes J. *Wonder Drug: The Secret History of Thalidomide in America and Its Hidden Victims*. New York: Random House; 2023.

85. Waggoner MR, Uller T. Epigenetic determinism in science and society. *New Genetics and Society*. 2015;**34**(2):177–95.

86. Fuller R, Landrigan PJ, Balakrishnan K, Bathan G, Bose-O'Reilly S, Brauer M, et al. Pollution and health: a progress update. *The Lancet Planetary Health*. 2022;**6**(6):e535–47.

87. Padula AM, Ning X, Bakre S, Barrett ES, Bastain T, Bennett DH, et al. Birth outcomes in relation to prenatal exposure to per-and polyfluoroalkyl substances and stress in the environmental influences on child health outcomes (ECHO) program. *Environmental Health Perspectives*. 2023;**131**(3):037006.

88. Kåks P, Målqvist M, Forsberg H, Fjellborg AA. Neighborhood income inequality, maternal relative deprivation and neonatal health in

Sweden: A cross-sectional study using individually defined multi-scale contexts. *SSM – Population Health*. 2025;**29**:101745.

89. Witt WP, Cheng ER, Wisk LE, Litzelman K, Chatterjee D, Mandell K, et al. Maternal stressful life events prior to conception and the impact on infant birth weight in the United States. *American Journal of Public Health*. 2013;**104**(S1):S81–9.

90. Cheng ER, Park H, Wisk LE, Mandell KC, Wakeel F, Litzelman K, et al. Examining the link between women's exposure to stressful life events prior to conception and infant and toddler health: the role of birth weight. *Journal of Epidemiology and Community Health*. 2016;**70**(3):245.

91. Harris ML, Hure AJ, Holliday E, Chojenta C, Anderson AE, Loxton D. Association between preconception maternal stress and offspring birth weight: Findings from an Australian longitudinal data linkage study. *BMJ Open*. 2021;**11**(3):e041502.

92. Hipwell AE, Fu H, Tung I, Stiller A, Keenan K. Preconception stress exposure from childhood to adolescence and birth outcomes: The impact of stress type, severity and consistency. *Frontiers in Reproductive Health*. 2023;**4**:1007788.

93. Sweeting JA, Akinyemi AA, Holman EA. Parental preconception adversity and offspring health in African Americans: A systematic review of intergenerational studies. *Trauma, Violence, & Abuse*. 2023;**24**(3):1677–92.

94. Rinne GR, Hartstein J, Guardino CM, Dunkel Schetter C. Stress before conception and during pregnancy and maternal cortisol during pregnancy: A scoping review. *Psychoneuroendocrinology*. 2023;**153**:106115.

95. Kasman AM, Zhang CA, Li S, Lu Y, Lathi RB, Stevenson DK, et al. Association between preconception paternal health and pregnancy loss in the USA: An analysis of US claims data. *Human Reproduction*. 2021;**36**(3):785–93.

96. Karlsson H, Merisaari H, Karlsson L, Scheinin NM, Parkkola R, Saunavaara J, et al. Association of cumulative paternal early life stress with white matter maturation in newborns. *JAMA Network Open*. 2020;**3**(11):e2024832.

97. Barker DJP, Osmond C. Infant mortality, childhood nutrition, and ischaemic heart disease in England and Wales. *The Lancet*. 1986;**327**(8489):1077–81.

98. Barker DJP, Osmond C, Forsen TJ, Kajantie E, Eriksson JG. Trajectories of growth among children who have coronary events as adults. *New England Journal of Medicine.* 2005;**353**(17):1802–9.

99. Figlio D, Guryan J, Karbownik K, Roth J. The effects of poor neonatal health on children's cognitive development. *American Economic Review.* 2014;**104**(12):3921–55.

100. Martinson ML, Reichman NE. Socioeconomic inequalities in low birth weight in the United States, the United Kingdom, Canada, and Australia. *American Journal of Public Health.* 2016;**106**(4):748–54.

101. Hines CT, Padilla CM, Ryan RM. The effect of birth weight on child development prior to school entry. *Child Development.* 2020;**91**(3):724–32.

102. Marsh J. *Class Dismissed: Why We Cannot Teach or Learn Our Way Out of Inequality.* New York: Monthly Review Press; 2011.

103. Declercq E, Zephyrin L. *Maternal Mortality in the United States: A Primer.* Issue Brief & Report. New York: Commonwealth Fund; 2020. (Available from: www.commonwealthfund.org/publications/issue-brief-report/2020/dec/maternal-mortality-united-states-primer.)

104. Thornburg KL, Boone-Heinonen J, Valent AM. Social determinants of placental health and future disease risks for babies. *Obstetrics and Gynecology Clinics of North America.* 2020;**47**(1):1–15.

105. Eskenazi B, Marks AR, Catalano R, Bruckner T, Toniolo PG. Low birthweight in New York city and upstate New York following the events of September 11th. *Human Reproduction.* 2007;**22**(11):3013–20.

106. Ohlsson A, Shah PS, Knowledge Synthesis Group of Determinants of Preterm/LBW births. Effects of the September 11, 2001 disaster on pregnancy outcomes: A systematic review. *Acta Obstetricia Et Gynecologica Scandinavica.* 2011;**90**(1):6–18.

107. Xiong X, Harville EW, Mattison DR, Elkind-Hirsch K, Pridjian G, Buekens P. Exposure to Hurricane Katrina, post-traumatic stress disorder and birth outcomes. *The American Journal of the Medical Sciences.* 2008;**336**(2):111–5.

108. Samari G, Catalano R, Alcalá HE, Gemmill A. The Muslim ban and preterm birth: Analysis of US vital statistics data from 2009 to 2018. *Social Science & Medicine.* 2020;**265**:113544.

109. Krieger N, Huynh M, Li W, Waterman PD, Van Wye G. Severe sociopolitical stressors and preterm births in New York City: 1 September 2015 to 31 August 2017. *Journal of Epidemiology and Community Health.* 2018;**72**(12):1147.

110. Legewie J. Police violence and the health of Black infants. *Science Advances.* 2019;**5**:eaax7894.

111. Entringer S, Buss C, Wadhwa PD. Prenatal stress, development, health and disease risk: A psychobiological perspective – 2015 Curt Richter Award Winner. *Psychoneuroendocrinology.* 2015;**62**: 366–75.

112. Webster P, Neal K. War and public health. *Journal of Public Health.* 2022;**44**(2):215–6.

113. Paul AM. *Origins: How the Nine Months Before Birth Shape the Rest of Our Lives.* New York: Free Press; 2010.

114. Hertzman C, Power C, Matthews S, Manor O. Using an interactive framework of society and lifecourse to explain self-rated health in early adulthood. *Social Science & Medicine.* 2001;**53**(12):1575–85.

115. Hertzman C, Boyce T. How experience gets under the skin to create gradients in developmental health. *Annual Review of Public Health.* 2010;**31**(1):329–47.

116. Karen R. *Becoming Attached: First Relationships and How They Shape Our Capacity to Love.* Oxford: Oxford University Press; 2024.

117. Hewlett BS, Winn S. Allomaternal nursing in humans. *Current Anthropology.* 2014;**55**(2):200–15.

118. Keller H, Chaudhary N. Is the mother essential for attachment? Models of care in different cultures. In: Keller H, Bard KA, eds. *The Cultural Nature of Attachment: Contextualizing Relationships and Development.* Cambridge: MIT Press; 2017. pp. 109–37.

119. Nelson CA, Fox NA, Zeanah CH. *Romania's Abandoned Children: Deprivation, Brain Development, and the Struggle for Recovery.* Cambridge: Harvard University Press; 2014.

120. Ehrlich KB, Cassidy J. Early attachment and later physical health. In: Thompson RA, Simpson JA, Berlin LJ, eds. *Attachment: The Fundamental Questions.* New York: The Guilford Press; 2021. pp. 204–10.

121. Ciechanowski P, Russo J, Katon WJ, Lin EHB, Ludman E, Heckbert S, et al. Relationship styles and mortality in patients with diabetes. *Diabetes Care.* 2010;**33**(3):539–4.

122. Felitti VJ, Anda RF, Nordenberg D, Williamson DF, Spitz AM, Edwards V, et al. Relationship of childhood abuse and household dysfunction to many of the leading causes of death in adults. The Adverse Childhood Experiences (ACE) study. *American Journal of Preventive Medicine.* 1998;**14**(4):245–58.

123. Raney JH, Weinstein S, Ganson KT, Testa A, Jackson DB, Pantell M, et al. Mental well-being among adversity-exposed adolescents during the COVID-19 pandemic. *JAMA Network Open.* 2024;**7**(3): e242076.

124. Felitti VJ, Anda RF. The lifelong effects of adverse childhood experiences. In: Chadwick DL, Alexander R, Giardino AP, Essemio-Jenssen D, Thackeray JD, eds. *Chadwick's Child Maltreatment: Sexual Abuse and Psychological Maltreatment. Volume 2.* Saint Louis: STM Learning; 2014. pp. 203–15.

125. Van der Kolk BA. *The Body Keeps the Score: Brain, Mind, and Body in the Healing of Trauma.* New York: Viking; 2014.

126. Adorno TW, Frenkel-Brunswik E, Levinson DJ, Sanford RN. *The Authoritarian Personality.* Norton paperback ed. New York: Harper; 1950.

127. Milburn MA, Conrad SD, Sala F, Carberry S. Childhood punishment, denial, and political attitudes. *Political Psychology.* 1995;**16**(3):447–78.

128. Milburn MA. *Raised to Rage: The Politics of Anger and the Roots of Authoritarianism.* Cambridge: MIT Press; 2016.

129. Saxe G, Stoddard F, Courtney D, Cunningham K, Chawla N, Sheridan R, et al. Relationship between acute morphine and the course of PTSD in children with burns. *Journal of the American Academy of Child and Adolescent Psychiatry.* 2001;**40**(8):915–21.

130. Blanchflower DG, Oswald AJ. Unhappiness and pain in modern America: A review essay, and further evidence, on Carol Graham's happiness for all? *Journal of Economic Literature.* 2019;**57**(2):385–402.

131. Madigan S, Deneault AA, Racine N, Park J, Thiemann R, Zhu J, et al. Adverse childhood experiences: a meta-analysis of prevalence and moderators among half a million adults in 206 studies. *World Psychiatry.* 2023;**22**(3):463–71.

132. Hughes K, Ford K, Bellis MA, Glendinning F, Harrison E, Passmore J. Health and financial costs of adverse childhood

experiences in 28 European countries: A systematic review and meta-analysis. *The Lancet Public Health.* 2021;**6**(11):e848–57.

133. Narayan AJ, Lieberman AF, Masten AS. Intergenerational transmission and prevention of adverse childhood experiences (ACEs). *Clinical Psychology Review.* 2021;**85**:101997.

134. Schofield TJ, Lee RD, Merrick MT. Safe, stable, nurturing relationships as a moderator of intergenerational continuity of child maltreatment: A meta-analysis. *Journal of Adolescent Health.* 2013;**53**(4):S32–8.

135. Bahanan L, Ayoub S. The association between adverse childhood experiences and oral health: A systematic review. *Journal of Public Health Dentistry.* 2023;**83**(2):169–76.

136. Nelson CA, Bhutta ZA, Burke Harris N, Danese A, Samara M. Adversity in childhood is linked to mental and physical health throughout life. *BMJ.* 2020;**371**:m3048.

137. Tedeschi RG, Calhoun LG. Posttraumatic growth: Conceptual foundations and empirical evidence. *Psychological Inquiry.* 2004;**15**(1):1–18.

138. Tedeschi RG, Shakespeare-Finch J, Taku K, Calhoun LG. *Posttraumatic Growth: Theory, Research and Applications.* New York: Routledge; 2018.

139. Tedeschi P, Jenkins M. *Transforming Trauma: Resilience and Healing through Our Connections with Animals.* West Lafayette: Purdue University Press; 2019.

140. Meyer BD, Rosenbaum DT. Welfare, the earned income tax credit, and the labor supply of single mothers. *The Quarterly Journal of Economics.* 2001;**116**(3):1063–114.

141. Turner S, Posthumus AG, Steegers EAP, AlMakoshi A, Sallout B, Rifas-Shiman SL, et al. Household income, fetal size and birth weight: An analysis of eight populations. *Journal of Epidemiology and Community Health.* 2022;**76**(7):629.

142. Lu Y-C, Kapse K, Andersen N, Quistorff J, Lopez C, Fry A, et al. Association between socioeconomic status and *in utero* fetal brain development. *JAMA Network Open.* 2021;**4**(3):e213526.

143. UNICEF Innocenti Research Centre. *Innocenti Report Card 18: Child Poverty in the Midst of Wealth.* Florence: UNICEF; 2023.

144. Markovits D. *The Meritocracy Trap: How America's Foundational Myth Feeds Inequality, Dismantles the Middle Class, and Devours the Elite.* New York: Penguin Press; 2019.

145. Bezruchka S. Early life and the social determinants of health. In: Bryant T, ed. *Handbook on the Social Determinants of Health.* Cheltenham: Edward Elgar; 2025. pp. 93–111.

146. American Cancer Society. *Cancer Facts & Figures 2011.* Atlanta: American Cancer Society; 2012.

147. Adler A. *What Life Should Mean to You.* Boston: Little Brown; 1931.

148. Sherman R. *Uneasy Street: The Anxieties of Affluence.* Princeton: Princeton University Press; 2017.

149. Taylor A. *The Age of Insecurity: Coming Together as Things Fall Apart.* Toronto: Anansi Press; 2023.

150. Easterlin R. Will raising the incomes of all increase the happiness of all? *Journal of Economic Behavior & Organization.* 1995;**27**(1):35–47.

151. Graham C. *Happiness Around the World: The Paradox of Happy Peasants and Miserable Millionaires.* Oxford and New York: Oxford University Press; 2009.

152. Marx K, Engels F. *The Communist Manifesto: A Road Map to History's Most Important Political Document.* Gasper P, ed. Chicago: Haymarket Books; 2005.

153. Wilkinson RG. Income distribution and life expectancy. *BMJ.* 1992;**304**(6820):165–8.

154. Kaplan GA, Pamuk ER, Lynch JW, Cohen RD, Balfour JL. Inequality in income and mortality in the United States: analysis of mortality and potential pathways. *BMJ.* 1996;**312**(7037):999–1003.

155. Kennedy BP, Kawachi I, Prothrow SD. Income distribution and mortality: Cross sectional ecological study of the Robin Hood index in the United States. *BMJ.* 1996;**312**(7037):1004–7.

156. Lynch JW, Kaplan GA, Pamuk ER, Cohen RD, Heck KE, Balfour JL, et al. Income inequality and mortality in metropolitan areas of the United States. *American Journal of Public Health.* 1998;**88**:1074–80.

157. Ross NA, Wolfson MC, Dunn JR, Berthelot JM, Kaplan GA, Lynch JW. Relation between income inequality and mortality in Canada and in the United States: Cross sectional assessment using census data and vital statistics. *BMJ.* 2000;**320**(7239):898–902.

158. Sanmartin C, Ross NA, Tremblay S, Wolfson M, Dunn JR, Lynch J. Labour market income inequality and mortality in North American metropolitan areas. *Journal of Epidemiology and Community Health.* 2003;**57**(10):792–7.

159. Auger N, Hamel D, Martinez J, Ross NA. Mitigating effect of immigration on the relation between income inequality and mortality: a prospective study of 2 million Canadians. *Journal of Epidemiology and Community Health.* 2012;**66**(6):e5.

160. Holt-Lunstad J, Smith TB, Layton JB. Social relationships and mortality risk: A meta-analytic review. *PLOS Medicine.* 2010;**7**(7):e1000316.

161. Wilkinson R, Pickett KE. *The Spirit Level: Why More Equal Societies Almost Always Do Better.* London: Penguin; 2009.

162. Chancel L, Piketty T, Saez E, Zucman G. *World Inequality Report 2022.* World Inequality Lab; 2021.

163. Diez Roux AV. The pervasive influence of wealth inequality on health. *JAMA Health Forum.* 2021;**2**(7):e211647.

164. Nettle D, Dickins TE. Why is greater income inequality associated with lower life satisfaction and poorer health? Evidence from the European Quality of Life Survey, 2012. *The Social Science Journal.* 2022;1–12.

165. Pickett K, Gauhar A, Wilkinson R, Sahni-Nicholas P. *The Spirit Level at 15.* London: The Equality Trust; 2024.

166. Pickett K. *The Spirit Level at 15 – Technical Appendix.* London: The Equality Trust; 2024.

167. Daly M. *Killing the Competition: Economic Inequality and Homicide.* New Brunswick: Transaction Publishers; 2016.

168. Rowhani-Rahbar A, Schleimer JP, Moe CA, Rivara FP, Hill HD. Income support policies and firearm violence prevention: A scoping review. *Preventive Medicine.* 2022;**165**:107133.

169. Weisheit R, Harmon MG, Ingram J, Cottle C. The geography of police killings utilising crowdsourced data. *The Howard Journal of Crime and Justice.* 2022;**61**(2):127–47.

170. Morgan S, Allison K, Klein BR. Strained masculinity and mass shootings: Toward a theoretically integrated approach to assessing the gender gap in mass violence. *Homicide Studies.* 2022;**28**(4):441–67.

171. Li S, Wu Z, Zhang Y, Xu M, Wang X, Ma X. Internet gaming disorder and aggression: A meta-analysis of teenagers and young adults. *Frontiers in Public Health.* 2023;**11**:1111889.

172. Kwon R, Cabrera JF. Income inequality and mass shootings in the United States. *BMC Public Health.* 2019;**19**(1):1147.

173. United Nations Development Programme (UNDP). *Human Development Report 2023/2024: Breaking the Gridlock – Reimagining Cooperation in a Polarized World.* New York: United Nations Development Programme; 2024.

174. Dewan P, Rørth R, Jhund PS, Ferreira JP, Zannad F, Shen L, et al. Income inequality and outcomes in heart failure: A global between-country analysis. *JACC: Heart Failure.* 2019;**7**(4):336–46.

175. Singh A, Peres MA, Watt RG. The relationship between income and oral health: A critical review. *Journal of Dental Research.* 2019;**98**(8):853–60.

176. Boyce JK, Klemer AR, Templet PH, Willis CE. Power distribution, the environment, and public health: A state-level analysis. *Ecological Economics.* 1999;**29**(1):127–40.

177. Hill TD, Jorgenson AK, Ore P, Balistreri KS, Clark B. Air quality and life expectancy in the United States: An analysis of the moderating effect of income inequality. *SSM – Population Health.* 2019;**7**:100346.

178. Montez JK, Grumbach JM. US state policy contexts and population health. *The Milbank Quarterly.* 2023;**101**(S1):196–223.

179. Nichols J. *Coronavirus Criminals and Pandemic Profiteers: Accountability for Those Who Caused the Crisis.* London: Verso; 2022.

180. Giridharadas A. *Winners Take All: The Elite Charade of Changing the World.* 1st ed. New York: Alfred A. Knopf; 2018.

181. Case A, Deaton A. *Deaths of Despair and the Future of Capitalism.* Princeton: Princeton University Press; 2020.

182. Loverock A, Benny C, Smith BT, Siddiqi A, Pabayo R. Income inequality and deaths of despair risk in Canada: Identifying possible mechanisms. *Social Science & Medicine.* 2024;**344**:116623.

183. National Academies of Sciences, Engineering, and Medicine, Harris KM, Majmundar M, Becker T, eds. *High and Rising Mortality Rates Among Working-Age Adults.* Washington, DC: The National Academies Press; 2021.

184. Sterling P, Platt ML. Why deaths of despair are increasing in the US and not other industrial nations – insights from neuroscience and anthropology. *JAMA Psychiatry*. 2022;**79**(4):368–74.

185. Rogers RG, Hummer RA, Lawrence EM, Davidson T, Fishman SH. Dying young in the United States: What's driving high death rates among Americans under age 25 and what can be done? *Population Bulletin*. 2022;**76**(2):1–31.

186. Ostry MJD, Berg MA, Tsangarides MCG. *Redistribution, Inequality, and Growth*. Washington, DC: International Monetary Fund; 2014.

187. Saez E, Zucman G. *The Triumph of Injustice: How the Rich Dodge Taxes and How to Make Them Pay*. New York: W. W. Norton; 2019.

188. Rostron A. The Dickey Amendment on federal funding for research on gun violence: A legal dissection. *American Journal of Public Health*. 2018;**108**(7):865–7.

189. Rosella LC, Kornas K, Negatu E, Zhou L. Variations in all-cause mortality, premature mortality and cause-specific mortality among persons with diabetes in Ontario, Canada. *BMJ Open Diabetes Research & Care*. 2023;**11**(3):e003378.

190. Todd E. *The Final Fall: An Essay on the Decomposition of the Soviet Sphere*. New York: Karz Publishers; 1979.

191. Bezruchka S, Namekata T, Sistrom MG. Improving economic equality and health: The case of postwar Japan. *American Journal of Public Health*. 2008;**98**(4):589–94.

192. US Surgeon General. *Smoking and Health: Report of the Advisory Committee to the Surgeon General of the Public Health Service*. Washington, DC: US Department of Health, Education and Welfare; 1964.

193. Cohen S, Doyle WJ, Baum A. Socioeconomic status is associated with stress hormones. *Psychosomatic Medicine*. 2006;**68**(3):414–20.

194. Sandi C. Stress and cognition. *Wiley Interdisciplinary Reviews: Cognitive Science*. 2013;**4**(3):245–61.

195. Carter CS. Oxytocin pathways and the evolution of human behavior. *Annual Review of Psychology*. 2014;**65**(1):17–39.

196. Taylor SE. *The Tending Instinct: How Nurturing Is Essential for Who We Are and How We Live*. New York: Times Books; 2002.

197. Carter CS, Kenkel WM, MacLean EL, Wilson SR, Perkeybile AM, Yee JR, et al. Is oxytocin "nature's medicine"? *Pharmacological Reviews.* 2020;**72**(4):829–61.

198. Zak PJ. The neurobiology of trust. *Scientific American.* 2008;**298**(6):88–95.

199. MacLean EL, Hare B. Dogs hijack the human bonding pathway. *Science.* 2015;**348**(6232):280–1.

200. Tryon MS, Stanhope KL, Epel ES, Mason AE, Brown R, Medici V, et al. Excessive sugar consumption may be a difficult habit to break: A view from the brain and body. *The Journal of Clinical Endocrinology & Metabolism.* 2015;**100**(6):2239–47.

201. Haushofer J, Fehr E. On the psychology of poverty. *Science.* 2014;**344**(6186):862–7.

202. Geronimus AT. *Weathering: The Extraordinary Stress of Ordinary Life in an Unjust Society.* New York: Little, Brown Spark; 2023.

203. Marmot M. *Status Syndrome – How Our Position on the Social Gradient Affects Longevity and Health.* London: Bloomsbury; 2004.

204. Marmot MG, Bosma H, Hemingway H, Brunner E, Stansfeld S. Contribution of job control and other risk factors to social variations in coronary heart disease incidence. *The Lancet.* 1997;**350**(9073):235–9.

205. Pereg D, Gow R, Mosseri M, Lishner M, Rieder M, Van Uum S, et al. Hair cortisol and the risk for acute myocardial infarction in adult men. *Stress.* 2011;**14**(1):73–81.

206. Sapolsky RM. *Why Zebras Don't Get Ulcers: The Acclaimed Guide to Stress, Stress-Related Diseases and Coping.* 3rd ed. New York: Henry Holt; 2004.

207. Driver EM, Gushgari AJ, Steele JC, Bowes DA, Halden RU. Assessing population-level stress through glucocorticoid hormone monitoring in wastewater. *Science of The Total Environment.* 2022;**838**:155961.

208. Ryan M, Gallagher S, Jetten J, Muldoon OT. State level income inequality affects cardiovascular stress responses: Evidence from the Midlife in the United States (MIDUS) study. *Social Science & Medicine.* 2022;**311**:115359.

209. Cohen S, Janicki-Deverts D, Chen E, Matthews KA. Childhood socioeconomic status and adult health. *Annals of the New York Academy of Sciences.* 2010;**1186**(1):37–55.

210. Shonkoff JP, Slopen N, Williams DR. Early childhood adversity, toxic stress, and the impacts of racism on the foundations of health. *Annual Review of Public Health.* 2021;**42**(1):115–34.

211. Blackburn EH, Epel E. *The Telomere Effect: A Revolutionary Approach to Living Younger, Healthier, Longer.* New York: Grand Central Publishing; 2017.

212. Lustig RH. *Metabolical: The Lure and the Lies of Processed Food, Nutrition, and Modern Medicine.* New York: HarperWave; 2021.

213. French SA, Tangney CC, Crane MM, Wang Y, Appelhans BM. Nutrition quality of food purchases varies by household income: the SHoPPER study. *BMC Public Health.* 2019;**19**(1):231.

214. Jones MJ, Goodman SJ, Kobor MS. DNA methylation and healthy human aging. *Aging Cell.* 2015;**14**(6):924–32.

215. Jung M, Pfeifer GP. Aging and DNA methylation. *BMC Biology.* 2015;**13**(1):7.

216. Kim S, Halvorsen C, Potter C, Faul J. Does volunteering reduce epigenetic age acceleration among retired and working older adults? Results from the Health and Retirement Study. *Social Science & Medicine.* 2025;**364**:117501.

217. Lu AT, Quach A, Wilson JG, Reiner AP, Aviv A, Raj K, et al. DNA methylation GrimAge strongly predicts lifespan and healthspan. *Aging (Albany NY).* 2019;**11**(2):303.

218. Gillman AS, Pérez-Stable EJ, Das R. Advancing health disparities science through social epigenomics research. *JAMA Network Open.* 2024;**7**(7):e2428992.

219. Krieger N, Testa C, Chen JT, Johnson N, Watkins SH, Suderman M, et al. Epigenetic aging and racialized, economic, and environmental injustice: NIMHD Social Epigenomics Program. *JAMA Network Open.* 2024;**7**(7):e2421832.

220. Gruenewald TL, Karlamangla AS, Hu P, Stein-Merkin S, Crandall C, Koretz B, et al. History of socioeconomic disadvantage and allostatic load in later life. *Social Science & Medicine.* 2012;**74**(1):75–83.

221. Kristenson M, Kucinskienė Z, Bergdahl B, Calkauskas H, Urmonas V, Orth GK. Increased psychosocial strain in Lithuanian versus Swedish men: The LiVicordia study. *Psychosomatic Medicine.* 1998;**60**(3):277–82.

222. Porges SW, Porges S. *Our Polyvagal World: How Safety and Trauma Change Us.* New York: W.W. Norton & Company; 2023.

223. Marya R, Patel R. *Inflamed: Deep Medicine and the Anatomy of Injustice.* New York: Farrar, Straus and Giroux; 2021.

224. Ranjit N, Diez-Roux AV, Shea S, Cushman M, Ni H, Seeman T. Socioeconomic position, race/ethnicity, and inflammation in the multi-ethnic study of atherosclerosis. *Circulation.* 2007;**116** (21):2383–90.

225. Vineis P, Delpierre C, Castagné R, Fiorito G, McCrory C, Kivimaki M, et al. Health inequalities: Embodied evidence across biological layers. *Social Science & Medicine.* 2020;**246**:112781.

226. Hegewald MJ, Crapo RO. Socioeconomic status and lung function. *Chest.* 2007;**132**(5):1608–14.

227. Mahmoud O, Granell R, Peralta GP, Garcia-Aymerich J, Jarvis D, Henderson J, et al. Early-life and health behaviour influences on lung function in early adulthood. *European Respiratory Journal.* 2023;**61**(3).

228. Gaffney AW, Himmelstein DU, Christiani DC, Woolhandler S. Socioeconomic inequality in respiratory health in the US from 1959 to 2018. *JAMA Internal Medicine.* 2021;**181**(7):968–76.

229. Ng M, Dai X, Cogen RM, Abdelmasseh M, Abdollahi A, Abdullahi A, et al. National-level and state-level prevalence of overweight and obesity among children, adolescents, and adults in the USA, 1990–2021, and forecasts up to 2050. *The Lancet.* 2024;**404**(10469):2278–98.

230. Global Obesity Observatory. Ranking (% obesity by country). World Obesity Federation; 2024. (Available from: https://data.worldobesity.org/rankings/.)

231. McLennan AK, Ulijaszek SJ. Obesity emergence in the Pacific islands: Why understanding colonial history and social change is important. *Public Health Nutrition.* 2015;**18**(8):1499–505.

232. Tanriover C, Copur S, Gaipov A, Ozlusen B, Akcan RE, Kuwabara M, et al. Metabolically healthy obesity: Misleading phrase or healthy phenotype? *European Journal of Internal Medicine.* 2023;**111**:5–20.

233. Richardson AS, Dietz WH, Gordon-Larsen P. The association between childhood sexual and physical abuse with incident adult severe obesity across 13 years of the National Longitudinal Study of Adolescent Health. *Pediatric Obesity.* 2014;**9**(5):351–61.

234. Popkin BM, Ng SW. The nutrition transition to a stage of high obesity and noncommunicable disease prevalence dominated by ultra-processed foods is not inevitable. *Obesity Reviews*. 2022;**23**(1): e13366.

235. Mazgelytė E, Mažeikienė A, Burokienė N, Matuzevičienė R, Linkevičiūtė A, Kučinskienė ZA, et al. Association between hair cortisol concentration and metabolic syndrome. *Open Medicine*. 2021;**16**(1):873–81.

236. Araújo J, Cai J, Stevens J. Prevalence of optimal metabolic health in American adults: National Health and Nutrition Examination Survey 2009–2016. *Metabolic Syndrome and Related Disorders*. 2018;**17**(1):46–52.

237. Noren Hooten N, Pacheco NL, Smith JT, Evans MK. The accelerated aging phenotype: The role of race and social determinants of health on aging. *Ageing Research Reviews*. 2022;**73**:101536.

238. World Health Organization (WHO) World Mental Health Survey Consortium. Prevalence, severity, and unmet need for treatment of mental disorders in the World Health Organization World Mental Health Surveys. *JAMA*. 2004;**291**(21):2581–90.

239. Kessler RC, Aguilar-Gaxiola S, Alonso J, Chatterji S, Lee S, Ormel J, et al. The global burden of mental disorders: An update from the WHO World Mental Health (WMH) Surveys. *Epidemiologia e psichiatria sociale*. 2009;**18**(1):23–33.

240. McGorry PD, Mei C, Dalal N, Alvarez-Jimenez M, Blakemore S-J, Browne V, et al. The *Lancet Psychiatry* Commission on youth mental health. *The Lancet Psychiatry*. 2024;**11**(9):731–74.

241. Morgan D, Grant KA, Gage HD, Mach RH, Kaplan JR, Prioleau O, et al. Social dominance in monkeys: Dopamine D-2 receptors and cocaine self-administration. *Nature Neuroscience*. 2002;**5**(2):169–74.

242. Alexander BK, Beyerstein BL, Hadaway PF, Coambs RB. Effect of early and later colony housing on oral ingestion of morphine in rats. *Pharmacology Biochemistry and Behavior*. 1981;**15**(4):571–6.

243. Lembke A. *Dopamine Nation: Finding Balance in the Age of Indulgence*. New York: Dutton; 2021.

244. Franchek-Roa K, Tiwari A, Lewis-O'Connor A, Campbell J. Impact of childhood exposure to intimate partner violence and other adversities. *Journal of the Korean Academy of Child and Adolescent Psychiatry*. 2017;**28**:156–67.

245. Slykerman RF, Thompson J, Waldie K, Murphy R, Wall C, Mitchell EA. Maternal stress during pregnancy is associated with moderate to severe depression in 11-year-old children. *Acta Paediatrica*. 2015;**104**(1):68–74.

246. Malaspina D, Corcoran C, Kleinhaus KR, Perrin MC, Fennig S, Nahon D, et al. Acute maternal stress in pregnancy and schizophrenia in offspring: a cohort prospective study. *BMC Psychiatry*. 2008;**8**:71–80.

247. Van den Bergh BRH, Marcoen A. High antenatal maternal anxiety is related to ADHD symptoms, externalizing problems, and anxiety in 8-and 9-year-olds. *Child Development*. 2004;**75**(4):1085–97.

248. Blazer DG. *The Age of Melancholy: Major Depression and Its Social Origins*. New York: Routledge; 2005.

249. Insel TR. *Healing: Our Path From Mental Illness to Mental Health*. New York: Penguin Press; 2022.

250. Harrington A. *Mind Fixers: Psychiatry's Troubled Search for the Biology of Mental Illness*. New York: W.W. Norton; 2019.

251. Moncrieff J, Cooper RE, Stockmann T, Amendola S, Hengartner MP, Horowitz MA. The serotonin theory of depression: A systematic umbrella review of the evidence. *Molecular Psychiatry*. 2023;**28**(8):3243–56.

252. Jablensky A. The 100-year epidemiology of schizophrenia. *Schizophrenia Research*. 1997;**28**(2–3):111–25.

253. Luhrmann TM, Dulin J, Dzokoto V. The shaman and schizophrenia, revisited. *Culture, Medicine, and Psychiatry*. 2024;**48**(3):442–69.

254. American Psychiatric Association. *Diagnostic and Statistical Manual of Mental Disorders: DSM-5-TR*. Washington, DC: American Psychiatric Association; 2022.

255. Watters E. *Crazy Like Us: The Globalization of the American Psyche*. New York: Free Press; 2010.

256. Twenge JM. *Generations: The Real Differences between Gen Z, Millennials, Gen X, Boomers, and Silents – and What They Mean for America's Future*. New York: Atria Books; 2023.

257. Haidt J. *The Anxious Generation: How the Great Rewiring of Childhood is Causing an Epidemic of Mental Illness*. New York: Penguin Press; 2024.

258. Office of the Surgeon General. *Our Epidemic of Loneliness and Isolation: The US Surgeon General's Advisory on the Healing Effects of*

Social Connection and Community. Rockville: Office of the Surgeon General; 2023.

259. US Department of Health and Human Services. *Mental Health: A Report of the Surgeon General.* Rockville: US Government; 1999.

260. Compton MT, Shim RS, eds. *The Social Determinants of Mental Health.* Washington, DC: American Psychiatric Publishing; 2015.

261. Nesse RM. *Good Reasons for Bad Feelings: Insights from the Frontier of Evolutionary Psychiatry.* London: Penguin Books; 2020.

262. Nesse RM. Anxiety disorders in evolutionary perspective. In: Abed R, St John-Smith P, eds. *Evolutionary Psychiatry: Current Perspectives on Evolution and Mental Health.* Cambridge: Cambridge University Press; 2022. pp. 101–16.

263. Strick LB, Ramaswamy M, Stern M. A public health framework for carceral health. *The Lancet.* 2024;**404**(10469):2234–7.

264. Mackenbach JP. Politics is nothing but medicine at a larger scale: reflections on public health's biggest idea. *Journal of Epidemiology and Community Health.* 2009;**63**(3):181–4.

265. Piketty T, Goldhammer A. *Capital and Ideology.* Cambridge: The Belknap Press of Harvard University Press; 2020.

266. Warren E, Tyagi AW. *The Two-Income Trap: Why Middle-Class Mothers and Fathers Are Going Broke.* New York: Basic Books; 2003.

267. Price CC. *Measuring the Income Gap from 1975 to 2023.* Working Paper WR-A516-2. Santa Monica: RAND; 2025.

268. Culpepper P, Shandler R, Jung JH, Lee T. "The economy is rigged": Inequality narratives, fairness, and support for redistribution in six countries. *Comparative Political Studies.* 2025;**58**(4):714–45.

269. Gilens M, Page BI. Testing theories of American politics: Elites, interest groups, and average citizens. *Perspectives on Politics.* 2014;**12**(03):564–81.

270. Barnes SG. *Waking the Sleeping Giant: Poor and Low-Income Voters in the 2020 Elections.* Washington, DC: Poor People's Campaign: A National Call for Moral Revival; 2021.

271. Montez JK, Mehri N, Monnat SM, Beckfield J, Chapman D, Grumbach JM, et al. US state policy contexts and mortality of working-age adults. *PLOS One.* 2022;**17**(10):e0275466.

272. Jacques O, Noël A. The politics of public health investments. *Social Science & Medicine.* 2022;**309**:115272.

273. Drutman L. *The Business of America is Lobbying: How Corporations Became Politicized and Politics Became More Corporate.* Oxford: Oxford University Press; 2015.

274. Tabery J. *Tyranny of the Gene: Personalized Medicine and Its Threat to Public Health.* New York: Alfred A. Knopf; 2023.

275. Bradley EH, Elkins BR, Herrin J, Elbel B. Health and social services expenditures: Associations with health outcomes. *BMJ Quality & Safety.* 2011;**20**(10):826–31.

276. Varoufakis Y. *Technofeudalism: What Killed Capitalism.* London: Bodley Head; 2023.

277. Pizzigati S. *The Rich Don't Always Win: The Forgotten Triumph over Plutocracy That Created the American Middle Class, 1900/1970.* New York: Seven Stories Press; 2012.

278. Harvey D. *A Brief History of Neoliberalism.* New York: Oxford University Press; 2005.

279. Rodríguez JM, Bae B, Geronimus AT, Bound J. The political realignment of health: How partisan power shaped infant health in the United States, 1915–2017. *Journal of Health Politics, Policy and Law.* 2022;**47**(2):201–24.

280. US Department of State. *Report by the Policy Planning Staff. PPS/23. Review of Current Trends: US Foreign Policy.* 1948. (Available from: https://history.state.gov/historicaldocuments/frus1948v01p2/d4.)

281. Carson-Parker J. The options ahead for the debt economy. *Business Week.* October 12, 1974. pp. 120–3.

282. Carey A. *Taking the Risk out of Democracy: Propaganda in the US and Australia.* Champaign: University of Illinois Press; 1997.

283. Crozier M, Huntinngton SP, Watanuki J. *The Crisis of Democracy: Report on the Governability of Democracies to the Trilateral Commission.* New York: New York University Press; 1975.

284. Warraich HJ, Kumar P, Nasir K, Joynt Maddox KE, Wadhera RK. Political environment and mortality rates in the United States, 2001–19: Population based cross sectional analysis. *BMJ.* 2022;**377**:e069308.

285. Jones CP. Levels of racism: A theoretic framework and a gardener's tale. *American Journal of Public Health.* 2000;**90**(8):1212–5.

286. Desmond M. *Poverty, by America.* New York: Crown; 2023.

287. Coates T-N. The case for reparations. *The Atlantic.* June 2014.

288. Robinson R. *The Debt: What America owes to Blacks.* New York: Plume; 2000.

289. Darity Jr WA, Mullen AK. *From Here to Equality: Reparations for Black Americans in the Twenty-First Century.* Chapel Hill: University of North Carolina Press; 2020.

290. Reeves A, Brown C, Hanefeld J. Female political representation and the gender health gap: A cross-national analysis of 49 European countries. *European Journal of Public Health.* 2022;**32**(5):684–9.

291. Vandemoortele J. The open-and-shut case against inequality. *Development Policy Review.* 2021;**39**(1):135–51.

292. Brady D, Kohler U, Zheng H. Novel estimates of mortality associated with poverty in the US. *JAMA Internal Medicine.* 2023;**183**(6):618–9.

293. Engels F. *The Condition of the Working Class in England in 1844.* New York: Lovell; 1887.

294. Galtung J. Violence, peace, and peace research. *Journal of Peace Research.* 1969;**8**:169–71.

295. Collins C, Flannery H. *Gilded Giving 2020: How Wealth Inequality Distorts Philanthropy and Imperils Democracy.* Washington, DC: Institute for Policy Studies and Inequality.org; 2020.

296. Flannery H, Collins C, DeVaan B. *The True Cost of Billionaire Philanthropy.* Washington, DC: Institute for Policy Studies; 2023.

297. Reich R. *Just Giving: Why Philanthropy Is Failing Democracy and How It Can Do Better.* Princeton: Princeton University Press; 2018.

298. Vallely P. *Philanthropy: From Aristotle to Zuckerberg.* London: Bloomsbury Publishing; 2020.

299. Schwab T. *The Bill Gates Problem: Reckoning with the Myth of the Good Billionaire.* New York: Metropolitan Books, Henry Holt and Company; 2023.

300. Domhoff GW. *Who Rules America? The Corporate Rich, White Nationalist Republicans, and Inclusionary Democrats in the 2020s.* 8th ed. New York: Routledge; 2022.

301. George H. *Progress and Poverty: An Inquiry into the Cause of Industrial Depressions and of the Increase of Want with Increase of Wealth.* New York: Appleton; 1886.

302. Estes R. *Tyranny of the Bottom Line: Why Corporations Make Good People Do Bad Things.* San Francisco: Berrett-Koehler; 1996.

303. Ludwig J, Duncan GJ, Gennetian LA, Katz LF, Kessler RC, Kling JR, et al. Neighborhood effects on the long-term well-being of low-income adults. *Science*. 2012;**337**(6101):1505–10.

304. Marmot MG, Davey Smith G. Why are the Japanese living longer? *BMJ*. 1989;**299**(6715):1547–51.

305. Franzini L, Ribble JC, Keddie AM. Understanding the Hispanic paradox. *Ethnicity & Disease*. 2001;**11**(3):496–518.

306. Reinhart E. Money as medicine – clinicism, cash transfers, and the political–economic determinants of health. *New England Journal of Medicine*. 2024;**390**(14):1333–8.

307. Kingdon J. *Agendas, Alternatives, and Public Policies (with an Epilogue on Health Care)*. 2nd ed. Harlow: Pearson; 2014.

308. Klein N. *The Shock Doctrine: The Rise of Disaster Capitalism*. New York: Metropolitan Books; 2007.

309. National Preventative Health Taskforce. *Australia: The Healthiest Country by 2020 – National Preventative Health Strategy – Overview*. Canberra: Commonwealth of Australia; 2009.

310. Rawls J. *A Theory of Justice*. Cambridge: Belknap Press of Harvard University Press; 1999.

311. Wiegmann DA, Wood LJ, Cohen TN, Shappell SA. Understanding the "Swiss cheese model" and its application to patient safety. *Journal of Patient Safety*. 2022;**18**(2):119–23.

312. Giridharadas A. *The Persuaders: At the Front Lines of the Fight for Hearts, Minds, and Democracy*. New York: Random House; 2022.

Index